ALSO BY CONSTANCE SANTEGO

FICTION
(Novels based on actual events)
The Nine Spiritual Gifts Series

Journey of a Soul - Companion novel to Archangel Michael

NONFICTION
The Intuitive Life, A Guide to Self-Knowledge & Healing through Psychic Development Second Edition

Fairy Tales, Dreams and Reality... Where Are You On Your Path? Second Edition

Your Persona... The Mask You Wear

Angelic Lifestyle – 42 Day Energy Cleanse

SECRETS OF A HEALER, SERIES:

    Magic Of Aromatherapy (Vol I)
    Magic Of Reflexology (Vol II)
    Magic Of The Gifts (Vol III)
    Magic Of Muscle Testing (Vol IV)
    Magic Of Iridology (Vol V)
    Magic Of Massage (Vol VI)
    Magic Of Hypnotherapy (Vol VII)
    Magic Of Reiki (Vol VIII)

Archangel Michael's Soul Retrieval Guide
Copyright © 2020 by Constance Santego.

All rights reserved. No part of this publication may be reproduced, distributed or transmitted in any form or by any means, including photocopying, recording, or other electronic or mechanical methods, without the prior written permission of the publisher, except in the case of brief quotations embodied in critical reviews and certain other noncommercial uses permitted by copyright law. For permission requests, write to the publisher, addressed "Attention: Permissions Coordinator," at the address below.

Copy Editor & Interior Design: Constance Santego
Book Layout: ©2017 BookDesignTemplates.com
Cover Design: Jennifer Louie

Ordering Information:
Quantity sales. Special discounts are available on quantity purchases by corporations, associations, and others. For details, contact the "Special Sales Department" at the address above.

Trade paperback ISBN: 978-1-7770818-0-5

eBook ISBN 978-1-7770818-1-2

Created and published In Canada. Printed and bound in the United States of America

First Edition
Published by Maximillian Enterprises
Kelowna, BC
Canada
www.constancesantego.ca

Archangel Michael's

SOUL RETRIEVAL GUIDE

Constance Santego

Maximillian Enterprises
Kelowna, BC

Dedication

To All my Students, Clients, and past Teachers.

Saint Michael the Archangel's Prayer

St. Michael the Archangel defend us in battle. Be our defense against the wickedness and snares of the Devil. May God rebuke him, we humbly pray, and do thou, O Prince of the heavenly hosts, by the power of God, thrust into hell Satan, and all the evil spirits, who prowl about the world seeking the ruin of souls. Amen.

Contents

Preface viii
Note to Reader x
Learning Outcome xi
Introduction 1
I Know Why Me 3
The Nine Spiritual Gifts 5
Are You Your Body? 13
Vibration & Destinations of the Spirit World 18
Destination Map 20
A Short Message from Archangel Michael 23
Soul Attachments 24
    How Do You Know If You Have an Attachment? ... 24
    Types of Attachments 27
    Test **ALL** Spirits! 32
How to Protect Against Spirit Attachments 34
    Protection Prayers 34
    Tools to Ward Off Negative Energy 41
    List of Spiritual Angelic Helpers 43
    Archangels vs Archdemons 46
    How to Call for the Help of an Archangel 52
    Meditation – Meet Your Angels 53
    Warrior Angel – Archangel Michael 61
    An Important Message Channeled from Archangel Michael 63
Removal of an Attachment - For Little Issues 65
    Induction A 67
    Induction B 69
    Induction C 70

    Induction D 72
    Creative Session #1 73
    Creative Session #2 77
    Creative Session #3 79
For Bigger Issues... 84
    Help from Archangel Michael 84
    Helping a Loved One/Ghost Ascend into Heaven 85
    Virtue and Deadly Sin Evaluation Test 89
    Choices in Heaven 92
    Creative Session #4 96
    Creative Session #5 98
    Creative Session #6 101
    Creative Session #7 104
    Creative Session #8 106
How Often Should You Clear Your Energy?........................ 108
Special Message From Archangel Michael 109
Bibliography... 111

Preface

Gift of Distinguishing Spirits

I was three the first time I remember seeing a ghost. By the age of eight, I knew how to close my eyes and never see them again. I grew up Catholic, and at the age of sixteen, after being to the Vatican City, and not fully understanding why the hoarding of riches when there were so many poor people in need, I decided religion was not what I believed it to be.

After hurting my back due to a work-related issue, I set out on a quest to heal myself. On my journey as being a natural health practitioner, spirits reappeared into my life, changing my beliefs of ghosts and the spirit world forever. I believe!

At the age of thirty-three, I magically owned a school. A few years later, it became an accredited college. After fourteen years, I opened a second school in Vancouver, B.C. Unfortunately, it bankrupted me, and I lost everything—even my faith and ability to see spirits.

I was devastated and embarrassed, not able to forgive myself. Not just because I went bankrupt, but because I didn't listen to spirit. I was told a year before to sell my college to my twenty-one-year-old daughter. It took seven years before I could hear spirit again.

Hindsight... I wish I had known better questions to ask my spirit guides.

Thank God, life goes on. I have a vision from when I was in my early thirties. I am on stage, speaking. It is an indoor amphitheater that can hold approximately eighteen-thousand people. It is packed. I am not sure what I am saying, but I can see what I look like. I believe this is going to happen. I do not know when, or how, or why. All I know is that I know I am speaking, and people are listening. This vision is what guides me every day of my life.

Today, I follow my instincts, pray... a lot, and listen to spirit, knowing I am not alone on my journey.

Enjoy your Journey, Constance

Note to Reader

This handbook is not to replace a medical doctor. It is a quick reference for Soul Retrieval. In many cases, I call upon Archangel Michael and the Bronze Master to assist me in removing a psychic attachment from a human.

To understand all that I am teaching, my suggestion to you is, read the companion novel 'Journey of a Soul' that compliments this manual.

Shift happens...Create magic!

Learning Outcome

When you have completed this manual and studied the concepts and techniques, you will be able to perform basic soul retrievals.

- Learn who to ask for help
- Learn the different types of attachments
- Learn how not to become a ghost
- Be able to perform a 'Soul Retrieval' for yourself, friends, or loved ones
- Learn how to get into Heaven
- Learn how to remove dark energy

Introduction

When a person becomes a lightworker – doing good for humanity, *your light attracts clients who need to feel better*. Students used to call my accredited natural health college, 'Magical.' Why? Because even though I was teaching a student, many modern techniques and modalities needed to become a Reiki Master, Natural Health, Holistic, or Spiritual Practitioner, the 'weird stuff' would happen.

Who knew that when you touch another person for longer than a few minutes that their life story is revealed, and not just because they told you about it? Many times, it came as a telepathic message or vision, or you could feel their pain in your body, or after they left, a strange feeling lingered in the room.

But what happens when your life-force energy is being drained, and it is not an innocent (harmless) client's energy that you are trying to rid?

Every day we are bombarded with negative energy, from computers, cell phones, TV's, microwaves ovens, automobiles, crime, food, drink, drugs, other people's negative moods, or pain that drains our life-force. So, why wouldn't you believe that invisible forces of evil spirits and demons could attach to you and devour your life-force energy, your light? Dark entities prowl on someone weak, sinful, vulnerable, and in need of help.

The old saying "like a moth to a flame" describes someone with an unswerving yet self-destructive attraction. Dark entities swarm to the light as a moth is drawn to a flame. This negative energy that swirls around a person who is in pain is what attracts dark entities, such as demons. To them, your life-force energy is the flame.

Essential oils, herbs, crystals, and prayer are a few examples of how to help you with healing subtle energy (physical, emotional, and mental). But when you need to heal spiritually, when you need help to protect you from a demon, you will need the power of Archangel Michael.

Through the help of Archangel Michael, I have created this guide that teaches you how to HELP yourself with a subtle energy crisis, or if you need help with a lost soul or beloved soul going home, or how to REMOVE dark energy attachments, energy vampires, and demonic spirits from a body.

In this guide, you will find the answers you were seeking.

I Know Why Me

I am on Earth to enjoy my last visit and to learn what I need to, for the memories are what I will keep when I die. These life lessons and all my experiences are vital for my job as an... *not sure if I get to call myself an archangel...* but for whatever I get to be called, I know I will be of service to humanity. I will make a difference if not on Earth, then from the Spirit world. *I will be bringing lost souls home.*

Summing Up What Is Waiting For You In The Afterlife?

- Know that whatever you believe is what is going to happen to you.
- Know ahead of time where you are going to go when you die! *Just have a demand and command! Or at least say, "I am going to the level of love-light energy (Heaven)."*
- Knowing that without a belief system, you can, unfortunately, become a ghost.
- Know that if you do not have a belief system in place, it may take many years, decades, or an eternity as being a ghost before you get help from a human who can sense you, to go into the light. *They cannot do it from Heaven! You had free will on Earth. They are honoring that wish!!!*
- Know that on your deathbed that you can ask for forgiveness, and it will be granted.

- Know that if you do not want to be, you will not be alone on the other side.
- Know that the spirit world is there to help you.

Now open your eyes... and Believe

The Nine Spiritual Gifts

In the New Testament, my favorite story is "The Gifts".
(Corinthians 1, Chapter 12, Verse 4-11)
(Maybe a little differently worded depending on which Bible you have).

The variety and the unity of gifts
There are many different gifts, but it is always the same Spirit; there are many different ways of serving, but it is always the same Lord. There are many different forms of activity, but in everybody, it is the same God who is at work in them all. The particular manifestation of the Spirit granted to each one is to be used for the general good. To one is given from the Spirit the gift of utterance expressing **wisdom**; to another the gift of utterance expressing **knowledge**; in accordance with the same Spirit to another, **faith**, from the same Spirit; and to another, the gifts of **healing**, through the same Spirit; to another, the working of **miracles**; to another **prophecy**; to another, the power of **distinguishing spirits**; to one, the gift of **different tongues** and to another, the **interpretation of tongues**. But at work in all these is one and the same Spirit, distributing them at will to each individual.

The New Jerusalem Bible

Following is an overview of the 'spiritual gifts.' What each gift is and how to develop each gift, is taught in my book, 'Secrets of a Healer – Magic of the Gifts.'
ISBN: 978-1-989013-07-6

Wisdom

Virtue & Deadly Sins
Ways to develop – Wisdom
- Akashic Records
- Meditation

Also, you can read my 'Secrets of a Healer – Magic of Hypnotherapy' book

Knowledge

Ways to develop – Knowledge
- Auras
- Astral Projection / Astral Travel
- Automatic Writing
- Past Lives
- Pendulum
- Psychometry

Also, you can read my 'Intuitive Life' book

Faith

The Maze
Ways to develop – Faith
- Prayer
- Reiki: Level 1 – The Apprentice

Also, you can read my 'Secrets of a Healer – Magic of Reiki' book

Healing

Ways to develop – Healing
- Secret of A Healer- Magic of (Aromatherapy, Reflexology, Massage, Hypnotherapy, Iridology, Muscle Testing & Reiki)
- Distance Healing – Energy Pool
- Chakras

Also, you can read my 'Angelic Lifestyles' book

Miracles

Ways to develop – Miracles
Also, you can read my Manifesting / Creating – 'Fairy Tales, Dreams and Reality' book

Prophecy

Ways to develop – Prophecy
- Energy & Psychic Readings

Also, you can read my 'Intuitive Life' book

Tongues

Ways to develop – Tongues
- Different Tongues
- Interpretation of Tongues
- Intuition

Also, you can read my 'Your Persona...The Mask You Wear' book

Distinguishing Spirits

Testing A Spirit
Ways to develop – Distinguishing Spirits
- Channeling/ Medium / Séance
- Spirit Guide/ Angel
- Mediumship
- A Loved One
- Séance – as a group
- Negative Energy
- Clearing a Build, Room, Place or Thing
- Release of an Entity / Removing Negative Spirits
- Removing negative energy using color meditation
- Removing negative energy using cord meditation
- Exorcism
- Bereavement / Grief

Also, you can read my 'Intuitive Life' book

Archangel Michael's

SOUL RETRIEVAL GUIDE

Are You Your Body?

Fascinating argument: Science has taught us facts that atoms are the basic units of matter and the primary structure of an element. We know that all matter is made up of atoms, and an atom is made up of three particles; electrons, protons, and nucleus – which are composed of even smaller particles such as quarks.

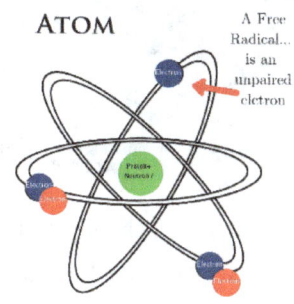

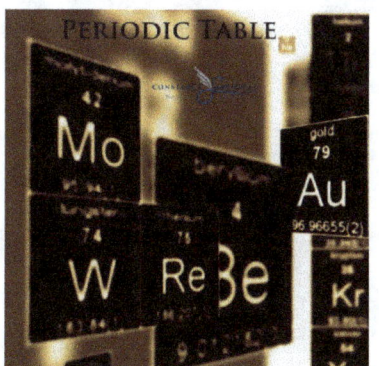

You might remember this from high school, there are 118 elements in the periodic table, which right now consist of 90 naturally occurring elements and the 28 man-made ones.

You might remember that protons and neutrons reside in the nucleus at the center of the atom and electrons exist in a cloud orbiting the nucleus, creating energy for the atom.

Part of my point is that if you add a proton to an atom, it makes a new element. And when atoms from different elements are joined together, forming compounds, they create molecules.

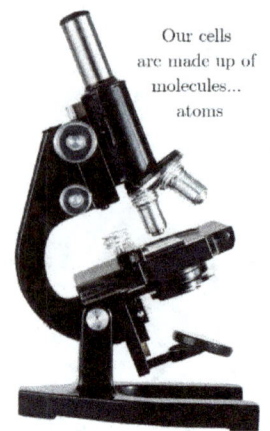

Our cells are made up of molecules... atoms

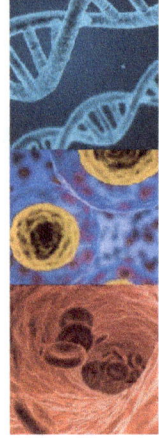

A human's eye is made up of molecules, as are a person's ears and the rest of their body. These molecules are made up of trillions of little atoms, and each of these atoms vibrates but stay fixed because of their strong attraction to one another.

I am getting to my point... molecules also create the paper and ink in a book that you are reading, the computer you may be watching, and even the steering wheel you might be holding! Everything a human can hear, smell, taste, touch or see in any of the four states of matter; solid, liquid, gas, or plasma are just trillions of tiny atoms creating our reality.

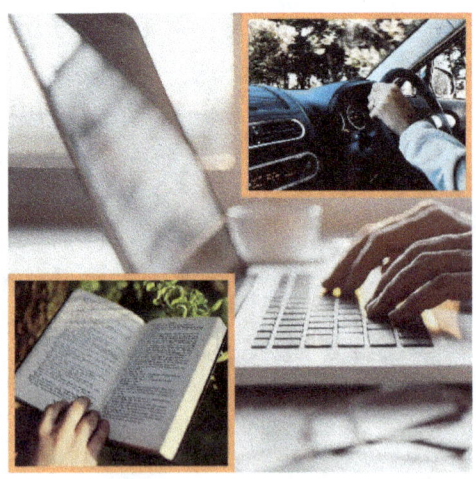

My guess is, that unless a person is taking a science class or is a scientist, every time they picked up a book, start typing on the computer or put their hands on the steering wheel, it never crossed their mind to think about what they were touching. . . minute atoms, vibrating so subtly the person cannot feel them.

There are many types of energy that can make a molecule move, such as mechanical, thermal, and chemical, to name a few.

Our world needs energy to function, as does our human body. We need the energy to stay alive, as in food, water, and air.

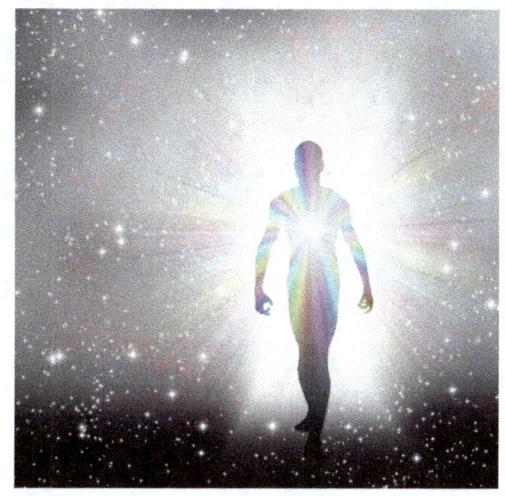

You use energy of light to read a book, and the potential energy as in a battery or electricity to be able to use a computer or to listen to a radio.

Our bodies are affected by the spectrum of electromagnetic energy, Radio Waves, TV waves, Radar waves, Heat, Light, Ultraviolet Light, X-rays, Short waves, Microwaves, and Gamma Rays.

Here is where I am going with this. All electromagnetic energy vibrates at a unique frequency, also known as hertz. My point is, atoms make up molecules, which creates matter, in this case, we are going to say a human body. And all matter has a frequency of vibration, in any state, solid, liquid, gas, or plasma.

Science has proven that when a human body dies, the original matter can all be accounted for except a minuscule amount of weight. This discrepancy is believed to be the SOUL that leaves the body. There is no scientific proof taught that a soul exists, but there is the fact of a weight issue at the time of death.

Are you your body?

You can stay alive without your arms, legs, some organs, even part of the brain, but you cannot stay alive without an energy flow of plasma—carrying blood, oxygen, and nutrients to all the cells needed for the function of your life.

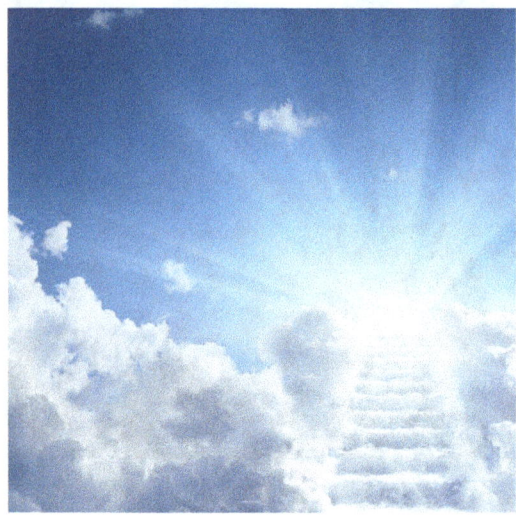

A scientist can create a lifeform by cloning a DNA carbon-based cell molecule ALREADY programmed for life. Meaning, scientists can only make a copy of the original, but they cannot make it from scratch. Without the program, a body will not work. By some miracle, a newborn baby's body is programmed with life and... a soul.

I believe... that a soul is a unique type of plasma, or some type of particle smaller than a photon or a fermion (an angel particle made of both matter and anti-matter), and faster than the speed of light, which has its own energy source and can access the human brain like the 'Matrix' creating our reality.

Are you your body?
I believe, Not.

I believe you are a soul.

***

What if we are a soul having a human experience?

Vibration & Destinations of the Spirit World

The lowest vibration of energy (not including animals and plants) are – **Humans,** we are the lowest level of energy that communicates with spirits. And, I am more scared of a human than the worst demon out there. Because humans have free will, meaning that they can do whatever they want to whenever they want to...

Ghosts are the next vibration of energy spirits. Ghosts are always, ALWAYS a lost soul. Meaning, after the person died, their soul never made it off Earth. Usually, this is due to the soul's belief or fear of the afterlife. In many cultures, religion has created a fear of where it will go to in the afterlife; Limbo, Purgatory, or Hell (or whatever name it is called in your belief system). And if a soul does not believe it can ascend into Heaven, it can choose to become a ghost and attach to a person, place, or thing on Earth.

The next level of vibration is called a **Spirit**; free moving souls, they can travel through time, dimensions, levels, and objects. This is the level that most people think of when they think of entities. As humans and ghosts can be good energy and bad energy - *yin and yang*, spirits can also be one or the other. There are many unique types of spirits, fairies, God, Devil, Demons, Archangels, and Saints like Jesus. Every spirit has a purpose, and for that reason, I am so thankful that the 'Spirit World' has very strict laws to protect us.

Destination

To me, the word dimension, level, and destination pretty much mean the same thing. No matter what name you use, I am writing about the vibration of atoms and the frequency of energy that an entity, anywhere, uses to exist.

Each destination is a unique frequency of energy. An entity that resides there shifts its vibration to resonate with that frequency.

Only spirits have the capability of free travel. Humans, ghosts, and lost souls do not have free travel. A human soul can astral travel, but it will always be like a dream. And ALL spirits have limitations to what they can do.

Destination Map

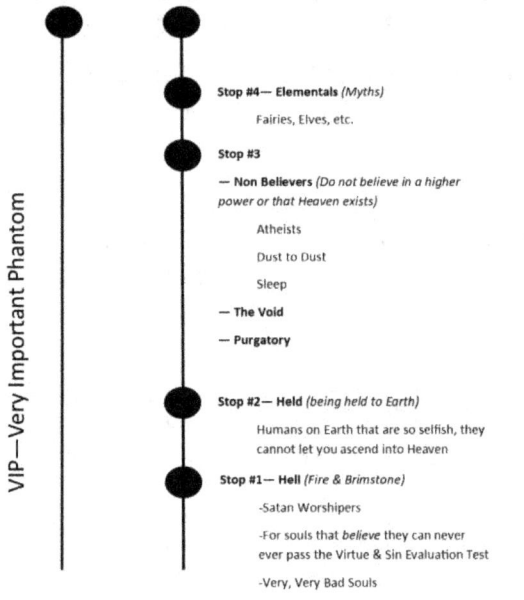

Destination Map — **Heaven**

Stop #5— Gates to Heaven *(Judgement Day—First Level of Heaven is Locked)*

Do you have the key to get in? First, Do you *Believe* in a higher power? Secondly, Did you pass the Virtue & Sin Evaluation test?

Stop #4— Elementals *(Myths)*
Fairies, Elves, etc.

Stop #3
— **Non Believers** *(Do not believe in a higher power or that Heaven exists)*
Atheists
Dust to Dust
Sleep
— **The Void**
— **Purgatory**

Stop #2— Held *(being held to Earth)*
Humans on Earth that are so selfish, they cannot let you ascend into Heaven

Stop #1— Hell *(Fire & Brimstone)*
-Satan Worshipers
-For souls that *believe* they can never ever pass the Virtue & Sin Evaluation Test
-Very, Very Bad Souls

VIP—Very Important Phantom

Train Station—*Limbo*

Earthly **Death** Choices:

1) Don't get on the train and become a Ghost—attach to a person, place or thing
2) Wait at the train station (in Limbo). This is for the agnostic, need more time, and just scared
3) Have a VIP Pass—Teleport instantly to the gates; First level of Heaven

Earth / Level of the Universe

The first destination is **HELL**
For Satan worshipers and for sinful souls that believe they deserve to be punished.

The second destination is **HELD**
For souls that are held and bound to Earth by a Human who is so selfish that they cannot let the soul ascend into Heaven.

The third destination is **NON-BELIEVERS**
For atheists, souls that do not believe in a higher power or that Heaven exists. For souls that believe they're just Dust-to-Dust or will go to Sleep. This third destination is also for souls going to the VOID or PURGATORY.
I want to mention that there is a special note that reads, with help from a Human Medium or Minister, a soul may have a chance for atonement.

The fourth destination is **ELEMENTALS**
For mythical souls, such as Fairies, Elves, Mermaids, etcetera.

The fifth destination is the **PEARLY GATES**
Express train for souls who believe in a higher power and are ready to take the Virtue and Sin Evaluation Test, or to be reincarnated.

The sixth stop and final destination is **HEAVEN**
For VIP - Very Important Phantom Ticket holders. Instant access through the Pearly Gates, no test required. While on Earth, the VIP soul or apparition must have

both entrance requirements. One, believe in a higher power of energy and two, lived a virtuous life."

Anyone who fails entrance into Heaven will stay
- in Limbo,
- or on Earth as a ghost, (your choice or could be destination two)
- or go to destination one or three

I have watched many movies filmed over the years portraying the spirit world. The stories that were written were based on so many similar experiences that I have had. But of course, Hollywood must portray the dead as scary so people can distinguish the difference between the living and the dead. I wonder what would happen if people knew how many movies and stories were based on facts and real experiences? Maybe, people would pay more attention to what they were watching on the big screen... or reading in a book.

Just as it is not safe to drive a vehicle without protection and training, it is not safe to conjure a spirit without protection and training.

Knowledge is Empowerment!

A Short Message from Archangel Michael

No entity or energy can enter your energy field without your permission. It may try and temporarily attach to you, but with prayer, aromatherapy, stones, talismans, herbs, blessed water, and other holy objects or objects of light, you can remove the attachment of energy.

Ask, and you shall receive.

Careful what you ask for, I only come when the energy is really needed.

Soul Attachments

How Do You Know If You Have an Attachment?

Entities can attach to a human soul when the soul is at a low point in its life; fear, depression, torment, foul moods, or when a soul is not in control of its body—operation, alcoholism, or drug use (medicinal or recreational).

When a person's energy is low or out of control, their energy field (auric field or vital field) becomes weak and develops cuts, holes, and distortions in the field. *The energy field is for protection, an outer layer of energy that emanates from every person like a shield or bubble.* If a field is not vibrating at one hundred percent, it can allow these dark forces and spirits the opportunity to attach to the person's soul or body, like a virus can when our immune system is not healthy.

In all cases, your life-force energy is being taken.

Symptoms or causes of having an attachment.
- You are a Light Worker, Healer, Psychic, or Natural Health Practitioners who are in other people's energy field.
- You dabble in the occult, Ouija boards, or spirit activities and do not have enough knowledge or training in esoteric or spiritual areas.

- There is paranormal activity such as noises, objects moving, seeing a presence
- You hear voices or an inner voice that continually criticizes you
- You practice satanic rituals or dark magic
- You have had a severe physical trauma
- You have had a head injury
- You have had surgeries or operations
- You feel as if you are being drained of energy, exhausted, constantly tired
- Bad things seem to happen to you, lots.
- You have a history of physical, emotional or sexual abuse (where personal power was lost)
- You get nightmares, terrifying dreams, sleep paralysis
- You have insomnia
- You have depression
- You have thoughts of suicide or homicide (thoughts of hurting yourself or others) that you cannot seem to stop
- You have done self-mutilation
- You have constant negative thoughts
- You get migraine headaches
- You are in any co-dependent relationships
- You have had unexplained forgetfulness or memory loss
- You get anxiety, panic attacks, phobias/paranoia,
- You have sudden changes in behavior or mood swings - irrational bouts of fear, anger, sadness or guilt
- You have addictive behaviors, including addiction to alcohol, drugs, cigarettes, sex, or gambling
- You have cravings or a major change in your eating habits
- you have a sudden weight gain or loss without a medical explanation
- You have impulsive behavior or have an attraction to dangerous situations

- You have an unexplained change in relationship problems
- You have felt like someone is watching you
- You have had an illness that will not respond to treatment or are of an unknown cause
- You have pain that does not go away and moves
- You have had a blood transfusion, organ transplant

Types of Attachments

There are many different types of attachments.

WALK-IN
Some spirits have ENTERED a body, and no one can remove it, no matter what they try to do, other than killing the person it now resides in. It is called a walk-in, also known as a soul transference.

A walk-in is a contract made in the afterlife with a nearly departed soul from Earth. At the time of death, the two souls exchange places. A new soul takes over the body and continues that life.

This new soul does not have to go through the years it took to get to that moment in time. It does not go through being a baby, learning all the things a body must know to function. Convenient if you ask me.

HOW TO RELEASE: You can't

SPIRIT POSSESSION
Is where a second soul (dark entity) ENTERS the body and can eventually take over. The first soul loses control over their body, speech, movement, how it dresses, and any other decisions. The original soul becomes tiny, taking up little space in the body and eventually dies.

Did you know that if you do not say a person's name when you are talking to them, you might not be talking to the person you think you are? If there are two or more souls in a body, the original soul can only speak if a direct question is asked by using their name. Other than that, the second soul is in control, convincing everyone that it is the original soul.

HOW TO RELEASE: Creative Session #8
You will ALWAYS need the help of Archangel Michael and the Bronze Master to remove these.

SOUL ATTACHMENTS

Some entities have ATTACHED themselves to a soul or body, but they do not reside in the body (as in possession or as in a walk-in). You probably don't even know that it is there. The attachment usually does not do anything to make you notice it. But it might cause you grief from time to time, especially if you know it is there and you do not get rid of it. Either way, if you notice it or not, the attached lost soul is stealing your life-force energy.

Soul attachments are very slowly stealing your life force energy, making you feel sick or causing you physical pain.

-Cords, Ropes, or Threads

Cords, ropes, or threads (thick or thin) can be attached to you from humans—also called an energy vampire (strangers, loved ones, friends, etc.), but can also be from dark entities.

HOW TO RELEASE: Creative Session #3
A chakra clearing meditation usually clears these.

-Demons, Dark Forces, Dark Entities, Moths, Reptilian, Mist, or Shadows

Fear and Negativity is the first thing they are attracted to. Also, unhealthy lifestyles, dark beliefs, emotions, and thoughts. Their mission is to cause misery and pain, to steal power, life-force energy, and the light of the people they possess.

HOW TO RELEASE: Creative Session #8
You will ALWAYS need the help of Archangel Michael and the Bronze Master to remove these.

-Elementals

An elemental is a spiritual being that belongs to one of the classic elements—fire, earth, metal, water, or air, and are impishly mischievous.

HOW TO RELEASE: Creative Session #3
Try a chakra clearing first, but you may need the help of Archangel Michael (Creative Session #6).

-Energetic Debris

We can pick up from other people. Traveling to new places, restaurants, night clubs, schools, the mall. Bad moods can become contagious.

HOW TO RELEASE: Creative Session #3
Do a chakra clearing meditation.

-Etheric Weapons

It can be from a present attack or past life, it can be how you died in a previous life, and the object was never removed (energy or residue imprints). Example: knife, bullet, rope, sword, or any other type of weapon.

HOW TO RELEASE: Creative Session #5
Do a removing etheric weapons meditation. You usually will not need the help of Archangel Michael.

-Holographic Inserts, Alien Implants
Light, chemical, emotional, mental, spiritual, or physical implants.

HOW TO RELEASE: Creative Session #8
You will need the help of Archangel Michael and the Bronze Master to remove any of these.

-Innocent Spirit Entities, Ghosts, Earth-Bound Spirits, Hauntings, or Poltergeists

These are human souls or fragmented souls. These attachments were human once, remember that! These souls are lost and need help going home.

HOW TO RELEASE: Creative Session #6
You may need help from Archangel Michael, but you may also be able to do the soul retrieval yourself.

-Incubus and Succubus

Demon sexual assault, alien-like with a tentacle that inserts into the body. Incubus (a demon in male form) inserts vaginally, and Succubus (a demon in female form) inserts orally.

HOW TO RELEASE: Creative Session #8
You will ALWAYS need the help of Archangel Michael and the Bronze Master to remove these.

-Spirit Attacks from Another Human

You will need to be clever and convince the entity that it is imprisoned, and to free itself. It needs to attack the one who sent it. Sometimes you need darker energy to get rid of dark energy.

HOW TO RELEASE: Creative Session #&
You will ALWAYS need the help of Archangel Michael and the Bronze Master to remove these.

-Soul Loss or Soul Fragmented

Is the loss of personal power from some traumatic experiences, which creates a parting of the soul, a piece of energy division from a person's aura.

HOW TO RELEASE: Creative Session #6
You may be able to do a chakra clearing, but you may need the help of Archangel Michael.

Soul Retrieval

Is an ancient healing method.

If the person is Alive: it can restore your lost personal power, or soul, and can close holes or openings within your energy field.

If the person is Dead: it can bring a soul home.

HOW TO RELEASE: Creative Session #4 or #6
Soul Retrieval Meditation. You may need the help of Archangel Michael and the Bronze Master.

Test **ALL** Spirits!

If you are removing an attachment, then you do not need to test the spirit.

BUT if you are going to LISTEN to a spirit, you need to test it!!! TEST even your angels and guides!!! Just take a moment to test it, no matter if you think it is a loved one like your mom, dad, grandma, etc.

The thought of love and light energy is powerful and purifying on its own, but it can be amplified by multiplying the amount of energy that you are aiming for. Many times, *I test the spirit three times* before I trust it. First, with just thinking love-light energy, then by amplifying the energy I am sending ten times, and then again by one hundred times the original love-light energy.

Once you trust and are familiar with the spirit you have communicated with, you will not need to test it each time.

PROCEDURE:

Imagine the spirit. Imagine sending love-light energy from your eyes and heart to the spirit's eyes and heart and hold that for a few moments. It usually only takes a few seconds to be rid of a low or dark spirit that has not had time to attach to you entirely (send the love-light energy for five minutes if you are unsure of how long). A low or dark spirit cannot handle the purifying power of the love-light energy. It will flicker or disappear in that amount of time.

1. Send love-light energy from your eyes and heart to the spirit's eyes and heart.
2. Hold for up to five minutes
3. Repeat - This time, send 10x the love-light energy from your eyes and heart to the spirit's eyes and heart.
4. Hold
5. Repeat - This time, send 100x the love-light energy from your eyes and heart to the spirit's eyes and heart.
6. Hold
7. If the spirit stays, you can communicate with it.
8. If it flickers and disappears. DO NOT TALK TO IT!

How to Protect Against Spirit Attachments

Have a healthy body, positive thoughts, and high vibration of energy.

If visiting the hospital, funeral home, or graveyard, protect yourself before you go. Wear an item (crystal, cross, crucifix, amulet) or pray. After, do a negative energy clearing.

Use Common Sense!

Protection Prayers

Prayers that I grew up with... words can be so powerful.

Constance Santego

> My own prayer that I say when I feel afraid or unsafe... *I believe in God; God is within me. Nothing can happen to God, so nothing can happen to me.*

Morning Prayer

> *In the name of our Lord Jesus Christ, I will begin this day. I thank you, Lord, for having preserved me during the night. I will do my best to make all I do today pleasing to You and in accordance with Your will. My dear mother, Mary, watch over me this day.*

My Guardian Angel takes care of me. St. Joseph and all you saints of God, pray for me...

Healing Prayer

Lord, you invite all who are burdened to come to you. Allow Your healing Hand to heal me. Touch my soul with Your compassion for others; touch my heart with Your courage and infinite Love for all; touch my mind with Your Wisdom, and may my mouth always proclaim Your praise. Teach me to reach out to You in all my needs and help me to lead others to You by my example. Most loving Heart of Jesus, bring me health in body and spirit that I may serve You with all my strength. Touch gently this life which you have created, now and forever. Amen.

"God grant me the serenity to accept the things I cannot change, courage to change the things I can, and wisdom to know the difference. Thy will, not mine, be done." Amen.

Meal

Before: *Bless us, O Lord! And these Thy gifts, which we are about to receive from Thy bounty, through Christ our Lord.*
Amen.
After: *We give Thee thanks for all Thy benefits, O Almighty God, Who livest and reignest, world without end. Amen*

Newly Departed Soul

May the souls of the faithful departed, through the mercy of God, rest in peace. Amen.

Saint Michael the Archangel

St. Michael the Archangel defend us in battle. Be our defense against the wickedness and snares of the Devil. May God rebuke him, we humbly pray, and do thou, O Prince of the heavenly hosts, by the power of God, thrust into hell Satan, and all the evil spirits, who prowl about the world seeking the ruin of souls. Amen.

The Chaplet or Divine Mercy

Recite on ordinary Rosary beads:
Begin with the Our Father, Apostle's Creed, and the three Hail Mary's.

Then on the large bead (Our Father bead) before each decade: *Eternal Father, I offer you the Body and Blood, Soul and Divinity of Your Dearly Beloved Son, Our Lord, Jesus Christ, in atonement for our sins and those of the whole world.*

On the ten small beads (Hail Mary beads) of each decade, say: *For the sake of His sorrowful Passion, have mercy on us and on the whole world.*

At the end of your Rosary (Say 3x): *Holy God, Mighty One, Holy Immortal One, have mercy on us and on the whole world.*

The steps to praying with a Rosary are (all prayers of the rosary are completed in a silent meditative state):

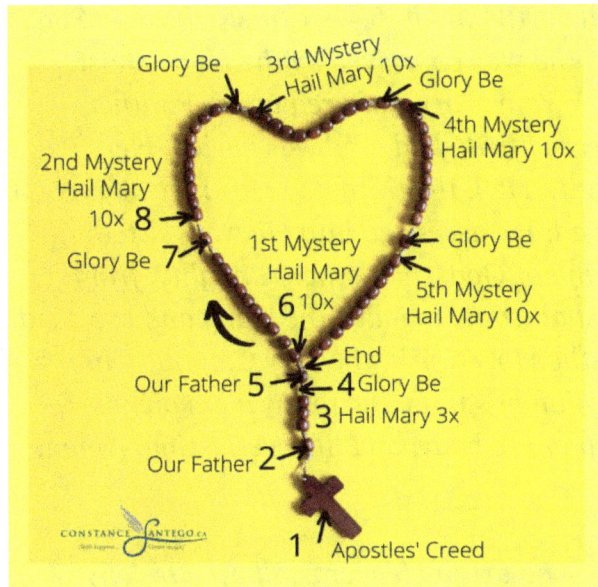

1. On the crucifix, make the sign of the cross, saying, "In the Name of the Father and of the Son and of the Holy Spirit," and then pray the 'Apostles' Creed.'
2. On the next *large* bead, say the 'Our Father' prayer,
3. On the following three small beads, pray three 'Hail Marys,' while meditating 'Faith, Hope, and Charity,'
4. On the *chain* or *cord,* pray the 'Glory Be' prayer,
5. On the large bead, meditate (intent or think) on the first mystery and pray the 'Our Father' prayer,
6. While meditating on the 2nd Mystery, on each of the ten (decades) beads, pray a 'Hail Mary' (one time each bead),
7. On the *individual bead,* pray the 'Glory Be' prayer,
8. Repeat Steps 5 thru 7 four more times to finish the next four decades and new mystery,
9. At the end of your Rosary, say the 'Hail Holy Queen' prayer,
10. Finish by making the "Sign of the Cross"

Apostles' Creed
> *I believe in God, the Father Almighty, Creator of Heaven and earth; and in Jesus Christ, His only Son, Our Lord, Who was conceived by the Holy Ghost, born of the Virgin Mary, suffered under Pontius Pilate, was crucified; died, and was buried. He descended into Hell; the third day He arose again from the dead; He ascended into Heaven, sitteth at the right hand of God, the Father Almighty; from thence He shall come to judge the living and the dead. I believe in the Holy Spirit, the holy Catholic Church, the communion of saints, the forgiveness of sins, the resurrection of the body, and life everlasting. Amen.*

Our Father
> *Our Father, who art in Heaven, hallowed be Thy name; Thy Kingdom come, Thy will be done on earth as it is in Heaven. Give us this day our daily bread; and forgive us our trespasses as we forgive those who trespass against us; and lead us not into temptation but deliver us from evil. Amen.*

Hail Mary
> *Hail Mary full of Grace, the Lord is with thee. Blessed are thou among women, and blessed is the fruit of thy womb Jesus.*
> *Holy Mary Mother of God,*
> *pray for us sinners now and at the hour of our death Amen.*

Glory Be.
> *Glory be to the Father, to the Son, and to the Holy Spirit, as it was, is now, and ever shall be, world without end. Amen.*

Hail Holy Queen.
> *Hail, Holy Queen, Mother of mercy, our life, our sweetness, and our hope. To thee do we cry, poor banished children of Eve, to thee do we send up our sighs, mourning and weeping in this valley of tears. Turn then, most gracious advocate, thine eyes of mercy toward us; and after this our exile show unto us the blessed fruit of thy womb Jesus, O clement, O loving, O sweet Virgin Mary.*
>
> *Pray for us, O holy Mother of God. That we may be made worthy of the promises of Christ.*
>
> *O God, whose only-begotten Son, by His life, death, and resurrection, has purchased for us the rewards of eternal salvation; grant we beseech Thee, that meditating upon these mysteries of the most holy Rosary of the Blessed Virgin Mary, we may imitate what they contain and obtain what they promise. Through the same Christ our Lord. Amen.*

Rosary Mystery's

There are five different mysteries to pray on, and each day of the week, the five mysteries change.

The **Five Joyful Mysteries** are traditionally prayed on Mondays, Saturdays, and, during the season of Advent, on Sundays:
1. The Annunciation
2. The Visitation
3. The Nativity
4. The Presentation in the Temple
5. The Finding in the Temple

The **Five Sorrowful Mysteries** are traditionally prayed on Tuesdays, Fridays, and, during the season of Lent, on Sundays:
1. The Agony in the Garden
2. The Scourging at the Pillar
3. The Crowning with Thorns
4. The Carrying of the Cross
5. The Crucifixion and Death

The **Five Glorious Mysteries** are traditionally prayed on Wednesdays and, outside the seasons of Advent and Lent, on Sundays:
1. The Resurrection
2. The Ascension
3. The Descent of the Holy Spirit
4. The Assumption
5. The Coronation of Mary

The **Five Luminous Mysteries** are traditionally prayed on Thursdays:
1. The Baptism of Christ in the Jordan
2. The Wedding Feast at Cana
3. Jesus' Proclamation of the Coming of the Kingdom of God
4. The Transfiguration
5. The Institution of the Eucharist

Tools to Ward Off Negative Energy

FOR LITTLE ISSUES

I have used Talismans before. Perfect for people who need to see or feel the protection (*Wiki: A **talisman** is an object that someone believes holds magical properties that provide power, energy, and specific benefits to the possessor*).

- Affirmations & Prayers
- Amber
- Amulets
- Belief in a higher power
- Cross
- Crystals (wearing or carrying hematite, black obsidian, smoky quartz, tiger eye, jet or black tourmaline)
- Coins, Gold & Silver
- Dragons
- Dream Catchers
- Essential Oils (frankincense, basil, camphor, eucalyptus, immortelle, many others)
- Faith
- Feathers
- Figurines - Buddha, Jesus
- Four Leaf Clover
- Garlic
- Holy Water
- Holy Wood (native to South America)
- Imagine a Protection Bubble or White Light around yourself

- Incense
- Laughter
- Light & Candles
- Lucky Rabbits Foot
- Mantra
- Night light
- Prayer
- Rosary
- Salt
- Security Blanket
- Smudge & Herbs (Sage and cedar)
- Sun & Moon
- Symbols
- Teddy Bear
- Totem Pole
- In the name of Jesus, I _____ _____
- Wood Carvings

List of Spiritual Angelic Helpers

Most people typically think of God or Jesus (son of God, he is for health, healing, and will greet you in Heaven) when they need emotional, physical, mental, or spiritual help.

Many people pray to a Saint for help (a Saint is a soul that walked on Earth as a Human and had accomplished three miracles before death).

- Saint Mary, Mother of Jesus, Motherhood
- St. Christopher, safe travels
- St. Patrick, help those in interpreting dreams and in following divine guidance
- St. Francis is the patron saint of animals and the environment
- St. Valentine, lovers, romance and of beekeepers and epilepsy
- St. Bernadette, of illness
- St. Anthony, lost things, lost causes, and most importantly lost souls.
- St. Augustine, of brewers and of those who struggle with a vice or habit they wish to break
- St. Joan of Arc, of soldiers, prisoners, captives, the Woman's Army Corps and France
- St. Padre Pio, civil defense workers, adolescents, and stress relief.
- St. Barbara's, tomb - site of miracles & of those at risk of sudden and violent deaths at work
- St. Gertrude the Great, to release the souls stuck in

purgatory
- St. Vincent de Paul, charities, volunteers, hospitals, prisoners & spiritual help
- St. Germain, is a legendary spiritual master of the ancient wisdom in various Theosophical and post-Theosophical teachings, responsible for the New Age culture of the Age of Aquarius – Ask for his violet flame

I have been introduced to four types of spirits that help us – **Guardian, Teacher, Worker,** and **Protector.**

The **Guardian Spirit's** job is to make sure we stay on our right path or life purpose. I have never known of a Guardian Angel to talk to us where we can hear them; they only direct us. We made our personal plans or life's purpose before being born into human existence, and it is the role of the Guardian Angel to see that we keep on track. Guardian Angels will not interfere with our choices unless they are against our personal plan or purpose.

A **Teacher Spirit** is who most people consider their guide. You might have one guide your whole life, or many, and they might change over the years. The role of these spirits is to teach us. They are with us most of the time, but not every day. These are the spirits that are the little voices in our heads telling us to do something. If the voice is directing us unwisely, we are being contacted by a low spirit or the dark side. Spirits of the light only want to improve life for everyone concerned.

Worker Spirits think they can still help, and in most cases, they can. They loved the job they were doing when they were alive so much that they want to continue helping others in the same field. They cannot change much of what is happening, but occasionally they leave us a message or give us extra energy when needed.

Protector Spirits do just that - they protect us when we are in harm. You might have heard stories of people avoiding disasters such as when a driver turns right instead of left, to find out later that he had missed involvement in a serious accident by turning at that moment.

Regardless of which spirit it is, you can ask any question you like. Actually, the more you learn about your personal spirit, the clearer your information or guidance will be. (Remember - test all spirits).

Many different religions have deities they pray to, find at least one you like and trust!

Here are some of the most well-known Archangels that you can ask for help:
- Archangel Michael, the Warrior Angel
- Archangel Raphael, the Healing Angel
- Archangel Gabriel, the Messenger Angel
- Archangel Ariel, the Angel of Nature and Animals
- Archangel Azrael, the Angel of Death
- Archangel Chamuel, Angel of Love & Peaceful Relationships
- Archangel Lucifer, Fallen Angel, and Ruler of Hell

Archangels vs Archdemons

An archangel is an angel of high rank, a chief angel in the celestial hierarchy. Archangels are powerful and divine beings who have exceptional abilities as healers and guides and intervene with assisting in many life's challenging situations.

Archdemons are also of high rank but are demonic beings who tempts us into sinful acts.

Fun fact – any angelic name ending in 'el,' means that the angel was never born a human.

Archangel/Virtue

Raphael	– Humility
Raziel	– Kindness
Azrael	– Patience
Gabriel	– Diligence
Michael	– Charity
Cassiel	– Temperance
Uriel	– Chastity

Archdemon/Sin

Lucifer	– Pride
Leviathan	– Envy
Satan	– Wrath
Belphegor	– Sloth
Mammon	– Greed
Beelzebub	– Gluttony
Asmodeus	– Lust

Archangel Ariel

Earth angel. Her name means 'lion or lioness of God,' and is the angel of environmentalism, nature, and animals. She assists in protecting, healing, rejuvenating, and maintaining our environment. Ask Archangel Ariel to help you protect the Earth, Universe, and creatures.

Archangel Azrael

Angel of Death. His name means 'Angel of God,' and is the angel of spiritual counseling. He assists ministers and spiritual teachers. Ask Archangel Azrael to help newly crossed-over souls adjust.

Archangel Cassiel

Tears angel. His name means 'Speed of God,' and is the angel of balance — yin and yang. He assists in the homeostasis (brings balance of the body, mind, and soul). Ask Archangel Cassiel for harmony within and without.

Archangel Chamuel – Gift of Knowledge

Peace angel. His name means 'he who sees God,' and is the angel of more profound vision and understanding. He assists you by protecting the world from fear and lower vibrating, negative energies. Ask Archangel Chamuel to find solutions to problems.

Archangel Gabriel – Gift of Tongues

Messenger angel and is a hermaphrodite. Its name means 'God is my strength', is the angel of communication. God's messenger. It assists writers, teachers, journalists, and artists to convey their message. Ask Archangel Gabriel to help you with your message.

Archangel Haniel

Moon Angel. Her name means 'Grace of God,' and is the angel of grace and joy. She assists anyone who seeks empowerment. Ask Archangel Haniel to help you develop your intuitive and healing abilities.

Archangel Hamied or Jesus – Gift of Miracles

Christ Light Angel. His name means 'Savior,' and is the angel of divine magic. They assist anyone who seeks help. Ask Jesus or Archangel Hamied to help you in times of need.

Archangel Jophiel

Creativity, Clarity, and Beauty angel. Her name means 'beauty of God,' is the angel of arts. She assists you in seeing and maintaining beauty in life, beautiful thoughts, creating and manifesting beauty. Ask Archangel Jophiel to help bring creative ideas.

Archangel Metatron

Recording Angel. He was born a human whom God transformed into an archangel. He assists anyone who seeks ascension and the ability to access spiritual powers. Ask Archangel Metatron to help you on your path to enlightenment.

Archangel Michael – Gift of Distinguishing Spirits

Warrior angel, his name means 'he who is as God,' and is the angel of protection, righteousness, mercy, and justice. He assists situations where you are afraid for your safety. Ask Archangel Michael to help you to cleanse space and for spirit releasement.

Archangel Raphael – Gift of Healing

Healer Angel. His name means 'God heals,' and is the angel of physical and emotional healing. He assists situations for the patient, client, or healer. Ask Archangel Raphael to help you cure addictions, cravings, injuries, and illnesses.

Archangel Ramiel

Hope Angel. His name means 'Thunder of God,' and is the fallen watcher angel. He assists you in true visions and is the watcher of the fallen angels. Ask Archangel Ramiel to guide you safely into Heaven.

Archangel Raziel – Gift of Wisdom

Secrets Angel. His name means 'Secrets of God,' and is the angel of mysteries. He assists you in bringing light into darkness. Ask Archangel Raziel to hear God's celestial and earthly messages and clear wisdom. To hear, see, feel, and know the secrets of the universe.

Archangel Sandalphon

Prayer Angel. Twin human brother to Metatron and believed to be the prophet, Elijah. Angel of music and musings. He assists you in bringing your prayers to God. Ask Archangel Sandalphon to bring the answers to your prayers (But be careful what you pray for).

Archangel Uriel- Gift of Faith

Faith Angel. His name means 'Light of God,' and is the angel of God's fire, inner strength. He assists you in granting strength for a spiritual battle within yourself. Ask Archangel Uriel to bring you love and gratitude.

Archangel Zadkiel

Patron Angel. His name means 'Righteousness of God,' and is the angel of freedom, benevolence, and mercy. He assists you in letting go of judgment. Ask Archangel Zadkiel to see the light in others.

Holy Spirit/Holy Ghost *aka* Bath Kol (Bat Qol)
– Gift of Prophecy

Voice of God. Her name means "Daughter of Voice,' is the angel of heavenly or divine voice that proclaims God's will or judgment. She assists in the will of God. Ask the holy spirit to bring you past, present, and future messages.

Archangel Lucifer – Fallen Angel

The story goes that Lucifer became so impressed with his beauty, intelligence, power, and position that he began to desire for himself the honor and glory that belonged to God alone. For this sin of pride, God cast Lucifer out of Heaven and made him Ruler of Hell. Guardian of Hell. He assists in bringing dark souls back to Hell and guarding sinful souls who end up there. Ask Archangel Lucifer to ward off demons and dark entities that have no right to your soul.

BE VERY SURE that a dark soul or demon is attacking you before invoking him. Ask God for help first. If the dark is needed to fight the dark, you will know.

Demons need to feed off life-force energy. When a person does even the slightest of sinful acts, this action gives way for a dark entity to feed, causing you pain and misery.

A new Demon is created only when a fully human soul descends into Hell, and that soul is so corrupt and evil that no punishment will ever save its soul.

How to Call for the Help of an Archangel

Just ask. You can pray, but all you need to do is ask for an archangel to come and help you to defeat an archdemon or to invoke your abilities and gifts.

When I ask archangel Michael to come and assist me, all I do is say, 'Archangel Michael, please come down and assist me with . . .'

ALWAYS when I am done with the task, I thank the angel who helped me.

Meditation –
Meet Your Angels

You can listen on my Constance Santego YouTube Channel —or have someone read it to you.

Meeting Your Angels and Guides

Close your eyes... get comfortable... get really relaxed... take a deep breath all the way down to the bottom of your lungs... Now let your breath out slowly and completely. Concentrate your attention behind your eyes... relax all the muscles in your eyes... relax them completely... relax them so much that they just don't open... breathing in and out slowly... relaxing even more... now take a deep, deep tummy breath... feel it as it expands every part of your lungs even more than the last breath... Now exhale slowly and completely... Let that same relaxation in your eye muscle go all the way down to your toes...let go completely... relaxing even more as you breathe in and out... all the way down to your toes.

Use your imagination... Now get ready to go beyond yourself... from this point on, let all outside noises increase your awareness of my voice... let my voice be your voice... relax your toes completely... adjusting your body whenever it needs to, to completely relax... concentrate all your attention in your feet... let go... all the muscles in your legs... concentrate on relaxing them now... your lower legs... and your upper legs... now concentrate on relaxing your hips... your lower abdomen... and your stomach... relax your lower back... let all the days, weeks built-up tension release from your entire back... every vertebra relaxing... not falling asleep... still very much aware of everything that is going on... able to hear my voice clearly... now relax all of the muscles in your shoulders and neck... relax your arms... all the way down to your fingertips... breathing in and out slowly and completely... relaxing even more, easier... even deeper... now concentrate on relaxing your face... your mouth... your cheeks... your jaw... your teeth... your forehead... relaxing your eyebrows... your ears... your hair...

...

You are very deeply relaxed now... not out of touch with reality... very much in tune with everything I am saying... completely aware of your surroundings... just very, very deeply relaxed... now you have reached a level of deep physical relaxation...

Let's concentrate on deep mental relaxation... for mental relaxation, I will count slowly from 100 to 98, so that you may double your relaxation with each number... when you reach 98, just let the numbers vanish. Here we go... 100... now double your relaxation, just let go... 99... double again your relaxation, now even more relaxed... 98... double one more time your relaxation... Now let the numbers vanish... Let them disappear... this is a nice stage of relaxation. Not out of touch with reality... deeply in tune with everything I am saying... completely aware of your surroundings... just very intent upon my voice... allowing all noises to increase your attention...very, very deeply relaxed...

Repeat mentally the following affirmation...

Each step I take is that much closer to my dream, wish, want and desire... I am unlimited...

I am so happy and grateful now that... I accept miracles in my life...

I am so happy and grateful now that... I am full of abundance in all areas of my life...

I am so happy and grateful now that... I am open to receiving infinite blessings from the universe...
I am so happy and grateful now that... I am successful in all areas of my life, and every day in every way I get better and better...

The next time you go into meditation, you will go even deeper... it will work even better... faster... deeper...

Now you will move to the higher side of yourself... pure spirit... a being of light... you are not your body... concentrate your attention on your toes... notice you have toes... and they are relaxed... but you are not your toes... notice your feet now... and your lower legs... and your upper legs... you are not these either... if you did not have your limbs, you would still exist... you are not your body... you are not your name... you can change your name and you are still you... notice your thoughts now... and you have thoughts... but you are not your thoughts... go even deeper now... give me your full attention... concentrate on my voice...

It is time to raise your vibrational rate with feelings of love and strong positive thoughts... you may do this by surrounding yourself with a beautiful protective white light... this white light represents truth... forgiveness... your ideal concept of the source, and all that is good... picture this white light now starting to glow in your heart... allow this white light to glow within your heart...

let it increase... feels its warmth and purity... allow it to extend and to radiate out of your heart so that it wraps around your body... completely surrounding you in a cocoon of pure white light... this white light is the source's perfect presence... you may actually see it, feel it, or sense it... but all you really have to do is to know it to be there... It will always be with you... you now have the protective white light around you so that your subconscious mind is only open to suggestions that are helpful and beneficial to you... bath yourself in the white light... notice you are light... unconditional pure love... pure compassion... pure forgiveness... you are beyond the beyond... you are one with the universe...
Breathing in...deep tummy breath... and relaxing... breathing out, releasing...
Enjoy this state of relaxation for a few more moments... take a few more deep breaths...
...

...

In a moment, I am going to ask you to experience yourself in a room, in the center of your head... behind your eyes... this room has doors that lead out of all sides... each of these doors leads to a guide or angel that you are destined to meet in this lifetime... a spiritual being on the other side... from the levels within Heaven... from the energy of love and light... I would like you now to imagine yourself in the room... Look around and experience all the doors... asking yourself which door you should open today... which guide or angel do you need to meet today... I want you to pick one door now... ask to experience the door in the most vivid form possible for you... you can see it... you can feel it... you can hear a description of it... or you can just know... how does it open...

On the other side of this door is your guide or your angel... or maybe even both at the same time... you can ask to have just one for today if you wish before you open the door... the most important one for your higher good will be there waiting for you, to greet you... not to worry, you can always come back and meet the others... we are going to make a conscious contract with your guides and angels... I want you to think about these three things after me...

My guides and angels have the highest level of integrity possible...

My guides and angels come in a form that I can easily accept...

My guides and angels are at the highest level that I can readily communicate with...

And anything else you would like to add that is specifically important to you...

...

Now notice the door you are standing in front of... open the door allowing your guide or angel to come in the most vivid form possible for you... so you can see it... feel it... know it... and hear it... greeting it in a way that feels comfortable... you can say hello... give it a hug... bow... shake its hand... you can ask it what its name is, or what you can call it... if it keeps changing its form, ask it to choose one shape...

Thank it for meeting with you...

Test the spirit... send love-light energy from your eyes and heart to the spirits eyes and heart...

Hold...

Send ten times the love-light energy from your eyes and heart to the spirit's eyes and heart...

Hold...

Send one hundred times the love-light energy from your eyes and heart to the spirit's eyes and heart...

Hold...

If the spirit disappeared, don't worry. When you try this meditation again, one will eventually stay. Continue to listen to this meditation, so that you know what will happen when you connect with a high energy angel or guide...

If the spirit remained...

Ask it what its responsibility is going to be in working with you...

...

Ask it how you are going to get the most out of your connection or time together...

...

Ask it how you can contact again in the future... and for what reason you can contact it in the future...

...

And anything else that you would like to ask...

...

...

...

I would like you now to get ready to say goodbye...

So, go ahead... saying goodbye... embracing them... shaking their hand... bowing to them... whatever seems appropriate... going back through the door... shutting the door behind you... Now, I want you to mark this door in some way so that you will always know that it leads to this guide or angel... you can put a symbol on it... you can write on it... anything at all.

...

In a moment, I am going to have you take another three deep breaths... as you breathe in, I would like you to envision that all your spiritual gifts are being awakened ... every cell right down to a DNA level awakening to this new level of awareness... as you breathe out, your intent is going to be to reprogram every cell down to the DNA to be attuned to this new level of quantum love and light energy...

So, breathing in that new level of spiritual awareness all the way down to the cellular level... breathing out, programming every cell down to the DNA to be filled with quantum love and light energy... breathing in that new level of spiritual awareness all the way down to the cellular level... breathing out, programming every cell down to the DNA to be filled with quantum love and light energy... one more time... breathing in that new level of spiritual awareness all the way down to the cellular level... breathing out, programming every cell down to the DNA to be filled with quantum love and light energy... knowing when you put your head down on your pillow tonight that you will fall asleep faster... sleep deeper... waking the next morning with even more vitality... with more inner peace... knowing your angels and guides are there to help you each and every day...

I am going to count from one to three... and when I get to three... you will be wide awake, fully alert, feeling wonderful... knowing that every cell has been attuned to quantum love and light energy... one, every cell down to the DNA has been attuned to quantum love and light energy... Two, it's a matter of allowing yourself to know that and to honor that... three, awake... wiggling your toes... stretching your arms... feeling wonderful... feeling so rejuvenated and alive...

Warrior Angel – Archangel Michael

Fact: Michael comes from Hebrew: / מִיכָאֵל
מיכאל (*Mīkhā'ēl* [miχa ' ʔel]), meaning "Who is like God?".

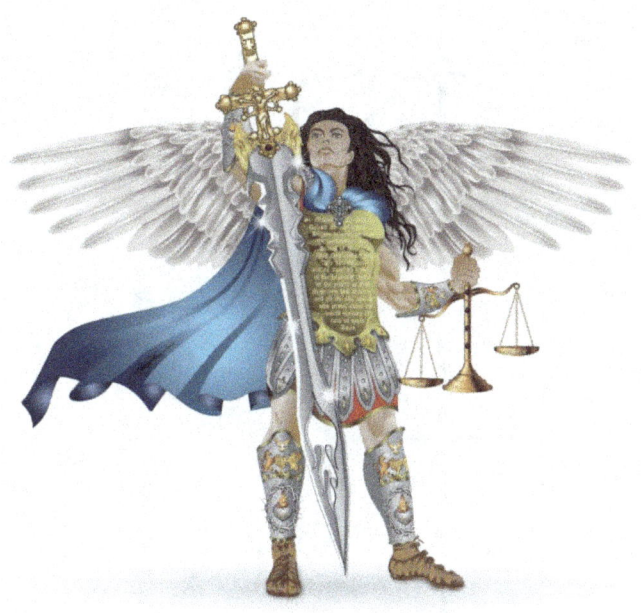

When I work on emotional, mental, spiritual, or physical issues like sore muscles, aches, and pains, it is only my knowledge of massage, crystals, aromatherapy, and healing that is needed.

Archangel Michael only comes to me when I am working on clients with dark energy or dark soul attachments.

If you look and read through the graph below, you will find that the big guns (God and Archangels) will only come out to help you when the energy is evil and way out of balance.

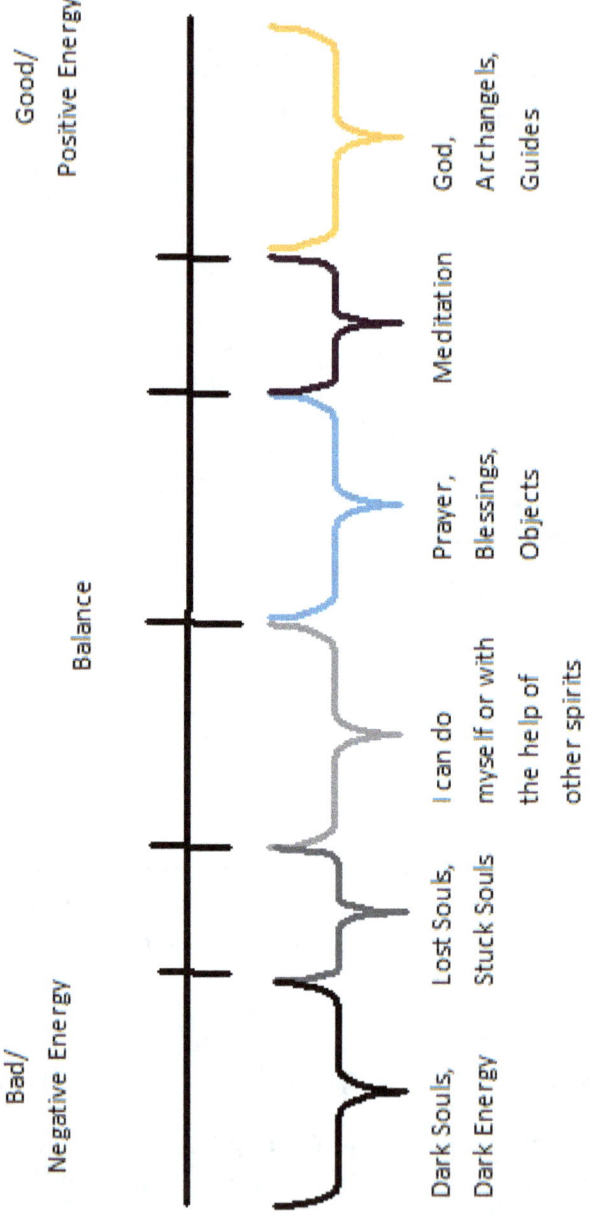

An Important Message Channeled from Archangel Michael

Dear loved ones, when you are asking to speak with your loved one that has passed on remember that you are asking to speak to someone who is dead to the materialistic world called Earth. The loved one no longer has a brain to create conscious thoughts and decisions. The loved one only has memories of the past, emotions of the past. I will not ask you how you are doing or feeling.

You have been given a blessing, a dream, a feeling, a voice, a thought to help you move forward in your own life, a message of peace, and gratitude of the loved one's wish for you when they were dying and still on Earth. My job as a messenger of God and a mover of spirits is one and the same. The message is this 'Dear ones. Please know that you are loved and that what waits for you on the other side is more of what you expect. Whatever you expect is what you will receive. There are many messengers that help to speak for us, like Constance. We call them, Earth Angels. You cannot understand us in the form we take, so we speak through those that have vocal cords, messengers that will do our service for us and help humankind on their life's journey on Earth.

Death is a scary word for many, the unknown, the void of existence. There are scary things on both sides of the veil that separates us from you. You have good people on Earth and bad people, and so do we. All have a purpose in balancing the universe and all levels of this domain. My message as a healer, no, that is Archangel Raphael. As a true messenger of God, no, the Holy Spirit and Archangel Gabriel and their troops do that work. My work as an angel of darkness, the angel that takes lost souls, lost entities, and dark spirits that are not welcome any longer, back home.

People like Connie, Constance, over the years has allowed me and my army of helpers to assist people that are burdened with dark energy and lost souls the gift of freedom, the gift of real magic, the gift of being in the light if they so choose. All souls and entities have the right to be in a better place. Ask, and you shall receive. The lost soul can't ask, so it attaches to someone that eventually and hopefully will seek the guidance of someone that has committed his or her life to help others. Take care and ask when you need help. Help will be on the way.

It will sometimes come in the most bizarre way.

Removal of an Attachment - For Little Issues

All the 'Creative Session' are while you are in a meditative state.

When to do a meditation. . . any time that you need to. Some people will only have to meditate once, and the pain or issue will be cleared forever. Where other people will need to repeat meditations over again due to their daily life recreating the cause of the pain or issue.

Following, you will read that I have four different inductions that you can use for any of the 'creative sessions.' An induction is to relax your body and prepare you for the action part of the meditation.

> *You can go to my Constance Santego YouTube channel to LISTEN to the meditations <u>or</u> you can have someone read them to you.*

What you will need:
- Time
- A quiet space, free of distractions
- A comfortable place to lie or sit. Some people fall asleep while meditating. You may want to sit
- Blanket, your temperature may drop
- Some people like soft, quiet background music

- Notepad and pen, some people like to journal their experience after they are finished

Procedure:

1st - Choose one of the four inductions.

2nd – Choose one of the eight creative sessions

TO RELAX YOUR BODY
AT THE START OF A MEDITATION

Induction A

Get yourself ready... get yourself ready to relax and go beyond your usual... allowing yourself to go into the beyond.

Taking a deep breath in and letting it out slowly... knowing that you can meditate and relax with your eyes open or closed... you can meditate in an alpha state... semi trans-state or even wide awake... fully conscious... you do it all the time... watching TV, listening to music, long-distance driving... on your way home... anytime you are not consciously active, you are in and out of the alpha state... meditating.

Letting go of all outside noises... or disturbances from others ... relax even more now... listening to my voice... being able to hear and understand me completely... knowing that your subconscious mind understands every word that I am saying...

Knowing that you can change your body's position at any time to be more comfortable... breathing in and releasing slowly...

You have the ability to imagine anything you would like... you have the magical ability to change any words I am saying into words that work even better for your personal benefit... you have the magical ability to change your body's temperature to always be comfortable... warmer or cooler... whatever you need... by just taking a deep breath in and releasing slowly... imagining adjusting your temperature like a thermoset... or imagining that you are listening to my voice from the location of your dreams... maybe you are on a tropical island... with a warm calming breeze... not falling asleep... fully aware of my voice...

So, let yourself go... making yourself more relaxed with every breath you take... breathing in and slowly out... taking an even deeper breath and allowing your breath to relax you even more...

Concentrating on my voice... never falling asleep... always able to understand what I am saying... but very, very deeply relaxed...

Induction B

Get yourself ready... to relax...

Get yourself very comfortable... Get ready to release any negative energy holding you back from your wishes, wants, dreams, and desires... When you are ready, you can close your eyes or if you prefer to keep them open, that is okay too...

Taking a deep breath in... all the way down to your toes... releasing... relaxing...

Deep breath... breathing in... and relaxing even more ... breathing out, becoming calm and peaceful...

Three more times... breathing in...deep tummy breath... and relaxing...breathing out... your environment is so tranquil...

Breathing in... imagine sparkling, vibrant creative energy... breathe out... you are releasing any negative energy that you do not need into a cosmic vacuum cleaner, a cosmic garbage can...

Wonderful... 1 more time... breathing in...deep, deep breath... and relaxing...breathing out releasing...

Concentrating on my voice... never falling asleep... always able to understand what I am saying... but very, very deeply relaxed...

Induction C

Close your eyes... and get comfortable... get really relaxed... take a deep breath all the way down to the bottom of your lungs... Now let your breath out slowly and completely...

Concentrate your attention behind your eyes... relax all the muscles in your eyes... relax them completely... relax them so much that they just don't open... breathing in and out slowly... relaxing even more... now take a deep, deep tummy breath... feel it as it expands every part of your lungs even more than the last breath... Now exhale slowly and completely... Let that same relaxation in your eye muscle go all the way down to your toes...let go completely... relaxing even more as you breathe in and out... all the way down to your toes.

Use your imagination... Now get ready to go beyond yourself... from this point on, let all outside noises increase your awareness of my voice... let my voice be your voice... relax your toes completely... adjusting your body whenever it needs to... to relax completely ... concentrate all your attention in your feet... let go... all the muscles in your legs... concentrate on relaxing them now... your lower legs... and your upper legs... now concentrate on relaxing your hips... your lower abdomen... and your stomach... relax your lower back... let all the days, weeks built-up tension release from your entire back... every vertebra relaxing... not falling asleep... still very much aware of everything that is going on... able to hear my voice clearly... now relax all of the muscles in your shoulders and neck... relax your arms... all the way down to your fingertips... breathing in and out slowly and completely... relaxing even more, easier... even deeper... now concentrate on relaxing your face... your mouth...

your cheeks... your jaw... your teeth... your forehead... relaxing your eyebrows... your ears... your hair... you are very deeply relaxed now... not out of touch with reality... very much in tune with everything I am saying... completely aware of your surroundings... just very, very deeply relaxed... now you have reached a level of deep physical relaxation...

Let's concentrate on deep mental relaxation... for mental relaxation, I will count slowly from 100 to 98, so that you may double your relaxation with each number... when you reach 98, just let the numbers vanish. Here we go... 100... now double your relaxation, just let go... 99... double again your relaxation, now even more relaxed... 98... double one more time your relaxation... Now let the numbers vanish... Let them disappear... this is a nice stage of relaxation. Not out of touch with reality... deeply in tune with everything I am saying... completely aware of your surroundings... just very intent upon my voice... allowing all noises to increase your attention...very, very deeply relaxed...

Induction D

Get yourself comfortable...and close your eyes when you are ready... take three deep breaths *(blow with your mouth open)* ... all the way down to your feet and toes... Imagine all your muscles relaxing...

Now, as you breathe in and out, your legs are relaxing...

Take another deep breath... all outside noise diminishes as you relax...

Focusing now on your stomach and tummy area... all of your muscles and organs are relaxing...

Your blood circulation is flowing perfectly, your lymphatic and immune systems are cleansing and healing... whatever system and wherever the issue is in your body, it is balancing as needed...

Take another deep breath...

Now your shoulders, arms, and hands relax...
You may be feeling lighter or some people feel heavier, whichever it is for you is perfect...

Your neck and head are relaxing, even your eyebrows, ears, and chin... every muscle in your body is relaxed and as you breathe, relaxing even more...

Breathing in and out... knowing that you are in control and have the power over your situation...

Creative Session #1

GOLDEN WHITE LIGHT MEDITATION
-WHEN YOU NEED EXTRA ENERGY

Procedure:
1. Lie down or sit comfortably.
2. Start with an induction (A-D).

Meditation:

3. Now imagine that you have a shower of golden white light energy pouring over your body. As this golden-white light energy bathes your body, you feel its vibrant healing energizing effects.

As you breathe in and out slowly, this beautiful energizing energy creates such a feeling of wellbeing in your body that you are smiling on the inside as well as the outside. Knowing your day is boosted with this positive healing energy on all levels of your being.

As the light energy of this shower revitalizes you, your skin starts to soak in this amazing vibrant healing energizing light energy. Each cell easily and happily eats the light as if it was food, food that nurtures your body, as well as your mind and soul.

Even your DNA and your RNA are rejuvenated as this light penetrates the cells of your body. Your stem cells know exactly where to go to heal; your brain cells are refreshed and amplified for more creative responses and have a greater attraction to infinite sources of abundance and prosperity... Your body instantly adjusts... balances and creates perfect homeostasis.

Notice with each breath you take this light is energizing each and every cell in your body right down to your DNA.

This special energy is there any time of the day or night that you need it to be. All you need to do is take a breath and imagine the shower of golden white light rejuvenating, strengthening, and energizing you.

I would like you to shift your attention now to a specific situation that you have today. It may do with your health, work, finances, your family, or maybe it is on finding love. No matter what comes to your mind, allow this thought to be what your subconscious mind; your inner genie needs to be working on today.

As the golden light touches your energy field and your body, your mind becomes more focused on finding a perfect answer to your situation. Everything becomes clearer, and as you ask this question, *"Inner Genie, please show me with a dream, words, feelings, or thoughts the perfect solution to my situation today."* Your subconscious mind instantly focuses on an answer.

...

As you take your next breath, your subconscious mind; your inner genie so easily adjusts to the question, the situation at hand and easily finds the answer, your solution for today's intent. Your inner genie is so happy that you are using the brilliance of your mind, the brilliance of infinite possibilities to assure that success will come forth into your life today.

Now that your body, mind, and soul are set to focus on bringing forth creative, healing, and success to your being, all you have to do is relax and receive the brilliant insights.

Your subconscious mind always focuses on what your emotions are feeding it. From now on you will nourish your subconscious this golden-white light energy to bring forth balancing and abundance of positive energy in every situation that arises in your life, knowing your subconscious mind, your inner genie has the power and ability to find the perfect solution.

Sending you in the perfect direction for your next step... It may be how to fix a situation, or it may be a new idea that will benefit your life, or it may guide you to an unexpected moment, and you find health, wealth, and happiness... every moment your inner genie is recalibrating and adjusting to your inner wishes, wants, dreams, desires, and goals.

As you ask, you shall receive...

As you practice bringing in this golden shower of energy, it becomes a habit, and automatically each morning as you awake to start your day, your inner genie will automatically turn on this shower of golden white light energy. It is always the perfect amount of revitalizing energy that you need to balance and harmonize your body, mind, and soul in every situation, every moment of your day.

Go forth with the empowering brilliance of your inner genie, knowing you can take a breath and get a perfect answer at any time that you need one.

...

In a moment you will coming back to the moment... knowing that you have this golden-white light energy which feeds vibrant healing energizing energy to each cell in your body, mind, and soul... with your next breath... wiggle your toes, coming back to the moment...

Creative Session #2

CLEARING OF BUILDING, ROOM, PLACE, OR THING MEDITATION

This technique is used when there is bad energy around a person. Great for clearing energy on vehicles, electronics, planes, houses, and many other items. There is only one rule; you can only do this creative session on anything or anybody that has a direct negative effect on you. You cannot do it on friends and family's belongings without their permission first. The same thing for strangers - if it is not in some way going to affect you negatively, then you cannot use this technique without everyone's permission.

Procedure:
1. Lie down or sit comfortably.
2. Start with an induction (A-D).

Meditation:

3. Now allow love-light energy to enter down through your crown chakra...

Allow grounding energy to enter up through your feet...

Imagine the rooms, place, or thing that you need cleared of negative energy ... start in one corner and imagine black material covering over the walls... ceiling... and floor... over the furniture and even people...

...
...
...

Once you have gone through all the rooms... hallways... yard... garage... let the material stay and absorb any bad energy...
...

Now go back and remove the material, and in place of it, imagine the color of gold over everything...
...
...
...

Once the dark is removed, the material evaporates... into a sparkle of energy like fireworks... now say out loud or in your mind, any positive words that you would like to have remain...

Wonderful... now take a breath, wiggle your toes and open your eyes... coming back to the moment

I have created protection energy stronger than just using positive words by imagining roses representing love light energy on each corner of my building. And, when I really thought it was needed, I have used gargoyles on each corner of my building... Hey, churches do it. It works!

Creative Session #3

CHAKRA CLEARING MEDITATION
- REMOVING NEGATIVE ENERGY, CORDS, THREADS, ELEMENTAL ATTACHMENTS, AND LOST OR FRAGMENTATED SOULS

An easy meditation to free most of the subtle dark energies attached to you.

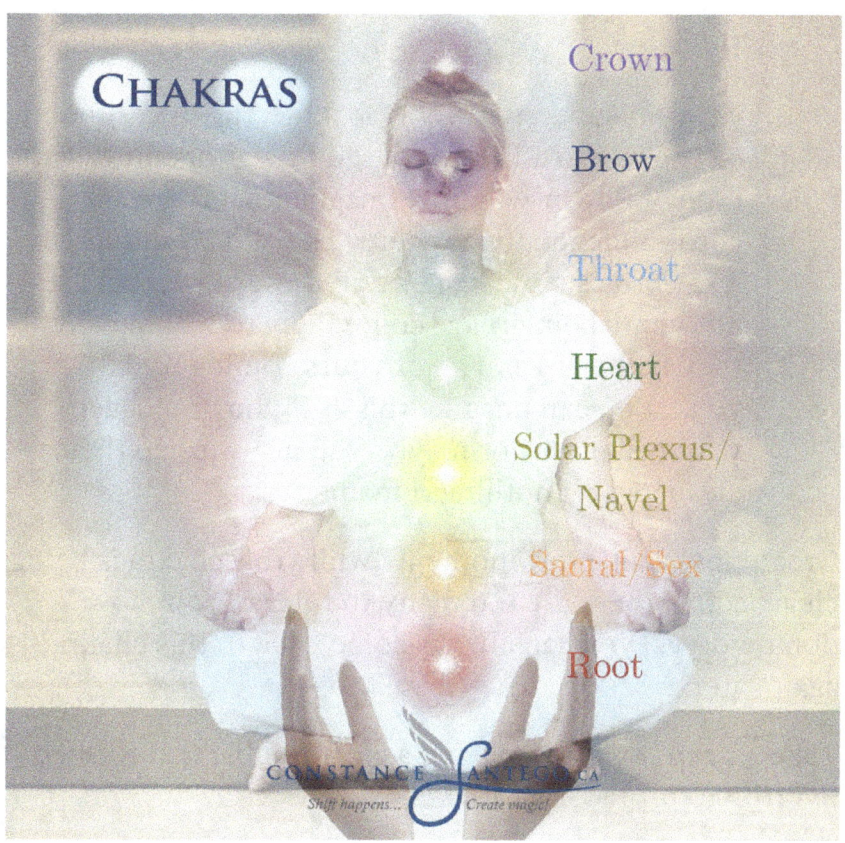

Many times, your life-force is being depleted due to energy vampires. These are humans that steal your energy. They can be friends, family, fans, and acquaintances that are the type of person who dominates an encounter. You will always know if this is happening because you feel exhausted after being with them for a half-hour or more.

Procedure:
1. Lie down or sit comfortably.
2. Start with an induction (A-D).

Meditation:

3. Now Imagine your Root Chakra... the lowest point of your torso... Imagine a red flower opening... any type of flower will do... Imagine that there are cords attached to you here. The Huna call these Aka cords... Now imagine all these cords that are not yours being released lovingly to whomever they belong to and all of yours coming back to you... You can imagine this as if you unplugged your cell phone or maybe you just washed them clean away... nothing remains...

Great, now wait a few moments while this chakra is being cleansed... if there are too many to release right now, don't worry... you can always come back to this chakra again later...

Take a deep breath... imagine a clear bubble that formed overtop to protect this area...

Now imagine your Sacral or Spleen Chakra... it is at the belly button... imagine an orange flower opening...

imagine releasing all the aka cords attached to you here... all of these cords that are not yours are being released lovingly to whomever they belong to and all of yours are coming back to you... Great, now wait a few moments while this chakra is being cleansed...

Again, if there are too many to release right now, you can always come back to this chakra again later...

Take a deep breath... and imagine a clear bubble overtop to protect this area...

With your next deep breath... imagine your Solar Plexus Chakra at the bottom of your sternum, where the ribs meet... imagine a yellow flower opening up... and these aka cords attached to you here are now being released... lovingly... all these cords that are not yours return to whomever they belong to and all of yours coming back to you...

It feels so wonderful to be cleansing your chakras ...

Take a deep breath... and imagine a clear bubble formed overtop to protect this area...

Next moving up to your Heart Chakra... located in the middle of your chest... it is a green flower that is opening... imagine all the aka cords are easily and effortlessly being released... lovingly to whomever they belong to... and all of yours comes lovingly back to you... take a deep breath... while this next chakra is being cleansed...

Breathing in and out... as you imagine that there is a clear bubble overtop to protect this area...

Moving up again... this time to your Throat Chakra... located at your throat... imagine a blue flower opening... and all the aka cords that are not yours being released lovingly to whomever they belong to and all of yours coming back to you.

Perfect, now wait again a few moments while this chakra is being cleansed...

Clear bubble...

Imagine your Brow or Third eye Chakra... between your eyebrows... it is an indigo flower that opens up... a cobalt blue... all of the aka cords go back to whomever they belong to... lovingly... and all of yours coming back to you...

One more left... now wait again while this brow chakra is being cleansed...

With your next breath... imagine the clear bubble overtop...

Imagine your Crown Chakra... spinning at the top of your head... at the baby soft spot... it is a violet flower that opens... imagine all the aka cords attached to you here... releasing all the cords that do not belong to you... lovingly going to whomever they belong to and all of yours coming back to you...

Take a deep breath... in and out... releasing...

Clear bubble...

Perfect, now that you have cleansed all the chakras, you will imagine... a beautiful crystal-clear light coming down from the heavens and entering down into your crown chakra, and this light flows all the way down your spinal column... and comes up through all the chakras... one by one... from the root chakra... right up through to the crown... this crystal clear light energy flows back out of your crown chakra like a water fountain and spills into your aura...

Imagine that your aura is only about three feet around you... above, behind, to the sides and below you... like a bubble...

This beautiful crystal-clear light continually cleans all the chakras... entering through your crown... flowing down over your spine... entering up through your root chakra... cleaning all the chakras as it flows up and out through your crown chakra again... and flows into your aura to cleanse it as well...

...

Now think positive words or affirmations... and imagine them being placed and vibrating in your cleansed aura...

...

Excellent...

Now take a deep breath and imagine this cleansed energy being sealed into your body and aura...

With your next deep breath... wiggle your toes and open your eyes, coming back to the moment...

For Bigger Issues

YOU MAY WANT TO GO TO A PROFESSIONAL

Psychic Medium
Priest or Minister
Shaman
Grand Reiki Master

If Not, try...

Help from Archangel Michael

These next creative sessions will help you understand how Archangel Michael assists in the battle against dark energy.

I am not usually told ahead of time if Archangel Michael is coming, I do not always know what type of energy I will be dealing with. Clients come in for all kinds of reasons—pain, confirmation, prediction, direction, and guidance.

Sessions start with, "What are you here for?"

Even though a client may book for a specific modality, it is not always the real reason they are coming to see me. Not every client says they are coming in to have negative energy removed from their body. But some of my favorite types of clients are the ones that have no idea why they are coming and just pray that I will address the issue accordingly, then the real magic can happen.

Helping a Loved One/Ghost Ascend into Heaven

These souls MUST go into the light. Freedom is waiting for them there, no more pain, anguish, fear, anxiety, no more negative emotions of any kind.

Some attachments are not what you think! Earth can be great, BUT only if you are alive. For a ghost Earth, is a prison.

If you feel, see, hear, or think of your loved ones daily then chances are they are not in Heaven they are stuck, lost souls here on Earth

Or worse yet, YOU are holding them here.

Imagine this...

I want you to sense the most vivid, beautiful energy that you can envision, now times that by a million, and that is what waits for you on the other side if you go into the light. All your loved ones that have passed on before you and that *have made it to the light* are there, your family, friends, and even your favorite animals. If you believe in Saints, Angels, Guides, and a God, they are all there waiting to greet you.

You have a choice in Heaven to do anything you wish for eternity. Many of you have an opportunity to be born again on Earth or be a walk-in and experience life through the body of other souls who are just departed.

I have been to funerals, and the soul that just passed on is floating around viewing from above. Sure, it can be one of their last wishes, and then they go into the light right after, but unfortunately, it is usually because they have become a lost soul and now can't go into the light on their own and attached themselves to someone or something at the funeral.

Help yourself first:

Before you die: If you do not already believe you are good enough to get into Heaven, then change your belief system.

If you do not believe in a higher power, then change your belief system.

And if not for you, then do it to help your loved ones go into the light.

After they die: Let the soul go from you - *What if your loved one is stuck now on Earth as a ghost, maybe for eternity... what happens when you die? They are still held here, and now you cannot reconnect with them in Heaven because they are not there.*

What you CAN do:

1. Let them go! Learn to forgive so that you are not the one that is holding your loved one here as a ghost.
2. Pray!
3. Pain medication can make a soul very disoriented, even if it believes in Heaven, so you may have to pray for their soul and make sure they are sent to Heaven.
4. Some people were really bad people, and made bad choices on Earth, pray for their soul to be taken to

the underworld, and cleansed of this negative energy so it cannot attach to a human and cause more pain.
5. Pray for your babies that died to be taken care of in Heaven.
6. Pray for yourself to be protected at the time of your death and taken to Heaven.
7. If they are on their death bed, pray to Jesus to take them to Heaven. There is power in your words. Jesus will come.
8. Envision them going into the love-light energy.
9. Imagine that a Heavenly Angel is coming to get them.
10. Imagine a conversation with them where their loved ones in Heaven are now with them reaching out their hands to grab them and bring them into the light with them.
11. Tell your loved ones on Earth to not fear your death and pray for you in Heaven and never be so selfish as to hold you down. Tell them to say it is okay and to go into the light.
12. If it was an accident, go to the site of your loved one's place of death and imagine sending their spirit home to Heaven. Or at least pray to Jesus or Archangel Azrael to bring them home to the light.
13. If it was a murder, pray for the soul to be at peace and go into the light. Pray for the soul to be released from the murderer's energy.
14. We do not know why all the souls have chosen to come and live a human life. It is not our job to judge other people's experiences. It is our job to send loving thoughts to the soul when it passes and make sure it goes into the light.

Just imagine a funeral, where instead of being sorry for OUR loss, we send love and light to the soul that just died. Imagine what would happen with a room full of that much love energy accumulating from the group and the impact on that soul. Imagine being in a room of that much love. It would be amazing! Heavenly!!!

I want you to know that if an entity removal was easy, then anyone could do it, and the stories of Priests doing exorcisms would not be heard of. My message to you is, don't fear the light and prepare yourself for the afterlife!

Don't become a lost soul!!!

I can help you while I am on Earth, but after you die, you will need the help of your loved ones WHO can sense that you have attached to them and then call me for the help of the Angels to guide your soul back home to Heaven.

*If you sense that you might have a loved-one attached to you, call on Archangel Michael to escort it home, into the light. If need be, seek professional help to help you send them home.

Virtue and Deadly Sin Evaluation Test

Virtue & Sin Evaluation Test

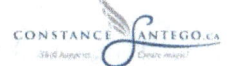

Focusing on Virtues; on a scale of 0% to 100%, write down the number that first comes to your mind with reference to the opposing Sin.

0% Bad ☀ ——————— ☀ 100% Good

Sin	Virtue	
Greed	Generosity/Charity	_____
Lust	Chastity	_____
Envy	Kindness	_____
Wrath/Anger	Patience	_____
Gluttony	Temperance	_____
Pride	Humility	_____
Sloth	Diligence	_____

Add All Virtues = Total _____

(Pass is 51% or better—add the total of all seven virtues and divide by 7) Mark _____ %

1st is the virtue of Charity or Generosity, which means kind, compassionate, and generous giving without expectation of anything in return. The opposite of Charity or Generosity is the deadly sin of Greed. Which is described as insatiability, materialistic, ravenousness, or voracity.

2nd is the virtue of Chastity. Which usually refers to refraining from any sexual conduct or romantic relationships, abstinence, and restraint. The opposite of Chastity is the deadly sin of Lust. Lust is described as an intensely powerful desire, craving, or yearning for a person, place, object, or circumstance.

3rd is the virtue of Kindness, which means having compassion, sympathy, thoughtfulness, or helpfulness towards someone in need. The opposite of Kindness is the deadly sin of Envy. Envy is described as wanting what another has with malice intent, resentment, ill will, or rivalry.

4th is the virtue of Patience. The state of endurance, tolerance, and persistence one has endured before negativity. The opposite of Patience is the deadly sin of Wrath or Anger. Wrath, rage, fury, madness is an emotional response to a perceived provocation, hurt, or threat.

5th is the virtue of Temperance, which is typically described as self-restraint, self-control, abstinence, or sobriety. The opposite of Temperance is the deadly sin of Gluttony. Which means excess, piggishness, over-indulgence in food, drink, or materialist items without having any control.

6th is the virtue of Humility. It is defined as being humble, obedient, modest, or unpretentious.

The opposite of Humility is the deadly sin of Pride, which refers to as gratification, arrogance, conceit, egotism, superiority, or any absurdly corrupt sense of one's vanity, value, status, or accomplishments.

7th is the virtue of Diligence. Diligent behavior is indicative of a work ethic; hardworking, industrious, and conscientious. The opposite of Diligence is the deadly sin of Sloth. Sloth is defined as lethargic, lazy, and reluctant to any type of exertion.

Choices in Heaven

Let my voice be heard on Earth, for when I am with the angels, you may not hear me anymore. I will still be there to help, but as a child of Earth, you may have shut your eyes and gone to sleep... *not able to hear me.*

No matter if it is you or your loved one who is afraid of dying or about to attach to a loved one... Here are some choices of what you can do or to tell a loved one to do when they get to the other side...

Options to think about before death. Will your choice be,

- To be reincarnated and live another life experience on Earth.
- To live in bliss and stay in Heaven for eternity.
- To live in bliss for as long as you wish to, and when your soul is ready, be reincarnated to live another life experience on Earth.
- To ascend to Nirvana – The only requirement is that you must have passed the enlightenment evaluation examination.
- Be reincarnated and live another life on a different planet.
- To live in bliss, and when your soul has accumulated enough life-experiences, evolve your soul on one of the seven levels of Heaven, or to choose one of the remaining eight levels in this realm, such as becoming an angel and helping humanity. Knowing that at any time, you have a choice of reincarnation and living the life you need to experience on Earth.
- Become a guardian angel and help others to stay on the right path in life.

- Become a protector angel and protect others from harm.
- Become a teacher angel AKA guide and help a soul on their journey through life.
- Become a worker angel and help others in their profession. An example is to imagine you are an airplane pilot, and after death, you help pilots who are in need.
- Become an animal spirit and help the animals.
- Become energy that helps the planet Earth itself.
- Become an assistant to another Saint, Angel or Archangel.

The more people who believe in the spirit world will create an evolution effect. Where new babies will grow up already knowing and never shutting their eyes to the truth, and so life and death will be that much easier.

Remember that you were born with free will; it is your choice on how you live your life, what you believe in, and what happens to you once you die.

TOP TWENTY RELIGIONS AS OF 2020

Christianity (2.1 billion) - Virtue & Sin test, all believe in an afterlife, and some believe in reincarnation.

Islam (1.3 billion) - Virtue & Sin test, believe you sleep or reincarnate, all believe in an afterlife.

Nonreligious (Secular/Agnostic/Atheist) (1.1 billion) - No belief in an afterlife.

Hinduism (900 million) / KARMA - Virtue & Sin test, all believe in reincarnation, and all believe in an afterlife.

Chinese traditional religion (394 million) - Virtue & Sin test, all believe in an afterlife or immortality.

Buddhism (376 million) - Virtue & Sin test, all believe in reincarnation, all believe in an afterlife and Nirvana.

Primal-indigenous (300 million) - Virtue & Sin test, all believe in an afterlife and a Great Spirit.

African traditional and Diasporic (100 million) – believe in a Supreme Creator.

Sikhism (23 million) - Virtue & Sin test, all believe in reincarnation, but believe there is no afterlife.

Juche – North Korean (19 million) – believe man is the master of his destiny.

Spiritism (15 million) - Virtue & Sin test, all believe in an afterlife, and that the soul can evolve.

Judaism (14 million) - Virtue & Sin test, all believe in reincarnation, and all believe in an afterlife.

Bahai (7 million) - Virtue & Sin test, all believe in an afterlife.

Jainism (4.2 million) - Virtue & Sin test, all believe in an afterlife and enlightenment.

Shinto (4 million) - Virtue & Sin test. Believe that the soul walks on Earth and helps their family and land to prosper.

Cao Dai (4 million) - Virtue & Sin test, all believe in reincarnation, all believe in an afterlife and Nirvana.

Zoroastrianism (2.6 million) - Virtue & Sin BRIDGE test; fall off, you go to purgatory for a re-test. Cross and you get an afterlife.

Tenrikyo (2 million) - Virtue & Sin test, Similar believes to reincarnation.

Neo-Paganism (1 million) AKA Wiccan - believe in an afterlife – also called Eternal Summer.

Unitarian-Universalism (800,000) – Science & Spiritual based, all blessings, and open to the idea Heaven might exist.

Creative Session #4

SPIRIT RELEASEMENT
-NEWLY DEPARTED SOUL

My cousin called me one day and said that a good friend of hers from high school has just passed. I knew of him; they were a year behind me. He was in his early fifties. She said he told her that he was not ready to die, that he still had plans. She was in town helping with his estate, and when going into the house, it felt icky, like something was wrong. She continued to tell me that another friend and her dog came with her, and at the entrance of the house, the dog started to make a funny noise and wanted in. Even the dog sensed something. Opening the door and letting the dog go free, the dog ran right to the spot where he had died.

She told me that she felt like the connection they had in life was lost, but she knew something was not right and called me to ask for my help.

> I proceeded to have her imagine him at any age. To imagine him and to direct him into the light, the love-light energy, I call it Heaven. To imagine his loved ones that have passed on before him or any animals that had passed on, to greet him and take him into the light with them.
>
> At that moment, both of us got tingles. Our bodies had shivers running up and down. It felt like his energy was ecstatic to leave the house and go to his loved ones in Heaven.

She was worried is soul was going to come back to the house. I told her not to worry, he is in the light now, that she did a great job. Not to worry, they could do anything with his possessions and the house, he was not attached to it any longer.

She said she wants to connect with him again, and I told her to wait a few days to give him time. Not to worry that she will be able to chat and connect with him very shortly after he adjusts to the love-light energy. *With some spirits, it's in seconds, but with others, it may take a few days.*

I thanked her for calling me to help him move on.

Creative Session #5

REMOVING ETHERIC WEAPONS MEDITATION

How you died in a past life can cause you pain and agony in this lifetime if the item was never removed from the body. For example, you were killed by a spear, arrow, rock, bullet, knife, water (drowning), poison or food blockage, plastic from suffocation, a tooth bite, metal or wood fragments, dirt, etcetera.

Procedure:
1. Lie down or sit comfortably.
2. Start with an induction (A-D).

Meditation

3. Great... now I want you to focus on any area in your body that there is pain, or uncomfortable or negative feelings or an issue...

If you have more than one area... start with one... we will continue to the next one later... think of a color... any color... the first one that comes to your mind... imagine that color as the pain... replace the pain with this color... focus on the color...

Now... imagine breathing in from the level of love and light... celestial energy coming in... a crystal-clear sparkly color... bring this new color in through the top of your head... the babies soft spot or crown chakra... all the way into the area of your pain...

Next, two things are going to happen...

First, if... there is an item from a past life that is still in this area... a cosmic doctor will appear and remove it... no need to fear this doctor... he or she is of the purest light... and is there to help you heal... allow the doctor to remove the item ... or items now... and whatever comes out goes into a cosmic incinerator... never to be used again... once all is removed... the doctor will heal this area... or areas instantly...

Second, no matter if there was an item or not... you are going to clean the area... imagine a vacuum cleaner attached to this area... and imagine bringing in the crystal-clear sparkly color energy down through your crown into the colored area... and allow the color to be pushed or pulled into the vacuum...

Do this until all the color is gone, and the crystal-clear sparkly color is left...

Take a nice deep breath...

Once the color is gone and the clear is left, create a new color, a healing healthy new color... first color that comes to mind... whatever color that is today...

Imagine this new color and have it come down through your crown and push the crystal-clear sparkly color out... so much color that the new color seeps into the vacuum...

Breathe...

Now think of as positive word or affirmation that you want to attach to the new colored area. An example might be, relaxation, free moving, energized, something to that nature... if you have more than one word... put in as many as you would like...

If you have more than one area that needs clearing, repeat the process... first color, removal if needed, crystal clear, and then the new color...

Breathe...

Once you have removed the bad energy... wiggle your toes and come back into your body... opening your eyes... feeling great.

Creative Session #6

REMOVING AN ATTACHMENT
-INNOCENT SPIRIT ENTITIES, GHOSTS, LOST SOULS, SOUL RETRIEVAL, EARTH-BOUND SPIRITS, HAUNTINGS, OR POLTERGEISTS, SOUL LOSS OR SOUL FRAGMENTED, AND ELEMENTALS

The word entity is another name for soul, ghost, or spirit, and it has a memory and can be scared. Many spirits and ghosts that are lost souls and have attached themselves to a human, just need help. Help to move on and into the light. Even dark spirits do not always know that they are captive to your body. All attached spirits or ghosts can only leave if they have help.

Client x comes in and has a session with me, and very quickly we find out that she has an entity attached to her... (*I can find this out when I ask if it has a name, and the client says, yes*).

Out loud, I ask... "Do you have a name?" (client answers). If yes, I take a breath and I **ALWAYS ask Archangel Michael to come down and assist me.** Then I continue with my questions...

"What is your name?" (client answers).
"Do you know where home is?"

    -If the client answers YES

"Would you like to go home now?" (if client answers yes). I say, "Archangel Michael, please bring this soul (spirit) home." And I take a breath and allow archangel Michael to take the soul home.

-If the client answers NO to any of these questions, *then this is where it gets interesting. I may have to be creative.*

*I must tell you another part of this story before I can keep going. I want you to imagine that you own a home, you love your home and everyone who lives in it. One day an army troop from who knows where (use your imagination) comes and tells you to leave. They are going to take over your property. What do you do, fight or flight?

This is the same problem an entity has of being forced out. No matter if it's because it's being kicked out or off, of a person, place, or thing, the spirit gets scared and has nowhere else to go, so it resists and fights back.

- If NO
I then ask, "Would you like to see where archangel Michael will be taking you?"
- If the client answers YES.
  I say, "Archangel Michael, please show this soul (spirit) where home is." I take a breath and allow archangel Michael to show the soul where it would be going. *Many times, once the soul sees where it will be going, leaps into its home all by itself.*

- If the client answers NO...
  I ask, "May I go with you and archangel Michael to see where you will be going? I promise you do not have to go if you do not want to." I take a breath and allow Archangel Michael to show us where it would be going. *Many times, once the soul sees where it will be going, leaps into its home all by itself.*

  If the soul does not like where it is going, I ask, "Archangel Michael, please show us another choice. *Many times, once the soul sees a place it likes, it leaps home all by itself (I don't have a better word to describe what happens, 'leaps' is the best description).*

  Many times, a soul/spirit will leave willingly as it sees a familiar face, loved one, or pet in the celestial home.

Rule #1 – While on Earth, have a belief in something more powerful than you and is of the light. *A spiritual being with the frequency of love-light energy.*
Rule #2 - Be Kind and Respectful to all entities. Most of them were human once.
Rule #2 - Speak with compassion and be polite!
Rule #3 – Do not assume.
Rule #4 – When in doubt, seek help!

If it still will not leave... go to Removing a Demon...

Creative Session #7

REMOVING A BONDED DEMON
- SPIRIT ATTACKS FROM ANOTHER HUMAN

A long time ago, I read a story in a book by Max Freedom Long. It goes something like this. It is about a man who went into the Hawaiian jungle and hired a group of locals to take him to a sacred area that many residents believed he was not permitted to go since he was a foreigner and had no permission to be going there.

On the trek, one of the guides became sick and was dying. Many in the group became scared and were about to run away. They feared that bad medicine or a voodoo curse was cast upon them, and none of them were safe if they kept helping this stranger. The foreigner said, "Wait, let me talk to this sick man first." He knelt and whispered into the sick man's ear.

I summon the energy that has cursed this man... Who has sent you?... Do you know why you are doing the bidding for the person that sent you?... Do you know by doing his bidding you are now captive and have accepted that he has control of you for the rest of eternity?... By the power invested in me, I release you now and demand you take with you the power of the curse and return it with full force onto the person who had you deliver it, and by doing this, you are free to leave and never serve that person again...

Within moments the sick man came alert and well. With amazement the group could not believe their eyes of the miracle which just took place. They traveled on to where the foreigner had paid them to journey, without another negative instance happening.

When they arrived back to their homes, they found out who the person was that had cursed their travels and that he had died while they were gone.

This story has given me so much inspiration to help the entities who were sent to attack or harm a human and help to free them from this bondage.

BUT, If the energy is dark and still does not want to leave...

I ask it if it knows that it is in bondage and cannot leave on its own?

I ask it many questions of how it came to be with that human and convince it that it will have freedom if it would move on.

It is up to Archangel Michael, where he takes the entity, not me. To have the entity leave the body easily, it must want to, and the human must want it to. Both must agree to want the same thing, to be gone, for it to leave. Either one can cause it to stay.

Again, in some cases, very few, I have witnessed an entity being removed without its approval. To help Archangel Michael, the Bronze Master, comes with his net and scoops up the soul with the removal of some of the darker entities, souls, and demons.

Creative Session #8

REMOVING A DEMON
DARK FORCES, DARK ENTITIES, MOTHS, REPTILIAN, MIST, OR SHADOWS, INCUBUS, SUCCUBUS, HOLOGRAPHIC INSERTS, AND ALIEN IMPLANTS

Living on Earth, there are corrupt and insane people who are never going to be of sound mind to make a morally correct decision. Think about prison, psychopaths, murders, rapists… no conscience, no remorse. Rare, but even the darkest lost souls have escaped the depths of Hell and have attached themselves to humans.

REMEMBER to treat every entity with respect and compassion. Our job is not to judge. It is to help bring the spirit home, wherever that is.

REMEMBER! Both the entity and human must agree to part ways. Make sure the human wants the entity gone and is not holding it from leaving.

If the client insists that the entity leaves his or her body…

And I've tried all the usual tactics, *remember the entity is scared and does not trust my words.* I invite it to allow me to travel with it to its home, spiritually. I tell it that Archangel Michael will show us its home, and if at that time it chooses not to stay, we will come back to the body it resides in.

Still, the spirit will not leave. . .

I have never had an entity that Archangel Michael determined irrational, not to be curious enough to go and have a peek at where home is. I am true to my word with the help of Archangel Michael. I also go to the spirit world of his home. Usually, we are greeted by his loved ones, and the entity instantly leaves Archangel Michael and me without hesitation. Sometimes it is a beloved animal that comes to welcome it and again poof it is gone from us.

Once in a blue moon, the entity has had to be shown a few places to choose from. I do not remember once where the entity who chose to take a peek, did not leave the body upon liking where it was going. It is always a better place than being attached to the human.

...Worst-case scenario, if I have tried everything and the spirit will not move on. I ask, "Archangel Michael, please bring the Bronze Master to remove this dark energy." The Bronze Master scoops up the dark entity, demon, moth, reptilian, mist, shadow, incubus, succubus, holographic inserts, alien implants with his net. And poof it is gone.

Spiritual Law - ONLY Archangel Michael can determine if the soul that is attached to the human is too corrupt that he has to override the entity's decision not to move on.

I know, so you are wondering why I don't just do that automatically? Let's imagine that you are the soul, and without your consent, poof, you are incinerated. No questions asked. Was it a fair trial? Did you get what you deserved? The same goes for the spirits. All souls were human. They deserve a chance for a better afterlife.

How Often Should You Clear Your Energy?

If you are not working with other people's energy as a career, playing with the occult, harming your energy field by abusing your body, visiting funeral homes, graveyards, or hospitals, you should hardly ever need help. BUT you can check as often as you like.

I usually do a chakra clearing and clearing of a building a couple of times a year.

I use a protection prayer or talisman as needed.

I only call Archangel Michael if it is extremely important!

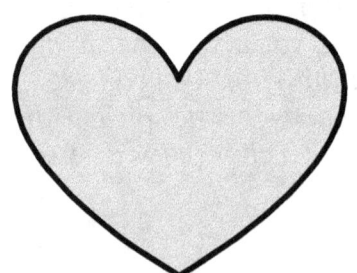

Remember, 'Love-Light Energy' is extremely powerful. Most of the time, that is all you will ever need!

Special Message From Archangel Michael

Here is what he said,

Even though Archangel Michael had come to help me many times, he never spoke. October 2019 was the first message I ever received from Archangel Michael.

You don't want to hear this; you are weak in mind and scared of the unknown. You are just a child in God's eyes, and you are so innocent. There is so much to tell and not enough time to speak the truth and give all the facts. You will know when it is your time to speak and the time to listen. Child of the Earth, please listen to what I must say, because there is so little time left before the next big crises. The crises of the wars of Heaven and Earth.

The crises of the time where energy is revealed, and all are awakened to know the true facts from Heaven, and where Earth is revealed in a new light. A light of darkness is awakened, and all souls are lifted to the light or removed from existence, and there is new energy revealed, and the truth of facts is eliminated because it will not matter anymore. Humans will not care that there was, at one time, a devil, or angels or even a God(s).

Humans will not care because the new revolution of energy will be so magnificent that all will be forgotten. Just like the new generations of today do not know what war is. Until one goes through the experience for themselves, it does not register or relate to real-time in a person's life.

You will know when it is time to listen and the time to speak. Energy is powerful, and when the masses, which are close, are of the same wavelength and frequency, energy changes. Just like in the experiments of quantum physics where energy when witnessed changes the pattern expected, so too will this new evidence of an energy that is so near to being revealed.

For now, all one can do is share your story and those that are ready will hear your message and know what to do with the evidence and start to share their experiences, and soon the message will spread to all parts of the world, and even the universe will sense the new frequency of energy of the masses. Like a stone dropped into an ocean, the wave travels on and on. The effect of the ripple is tenfold and four.

My message, for now, is simple... change your belief, and all is well.

What do you think his message means?

I find it interesting that a couple months later the Coronavirus crisis happened.

Bibliography

2007, The Intuitive Life, A Guide to Self-Knowledge & Healing through Psychic Development, under Connie Brummet

Archangel Michael

https://en.wikipedia.org/wiki/Michael_(archangel)

https://www.biblestudytools.com/topical-verses/archangel-michael-in-the-bible/

Celestial Languages
2017, In my book 'Your Persona... The Mask You Wear' I have written in more detail about the four channels of communication; audio, visual, knower and feeler.
ISBN:978-0-9952112-6-1

Prayers

https://www.catholic.org/prayers/popular.php

https://www.nursebuff.com/prayers-for-the-departed/

https://connectusfund.org/12-good-prayers-for-the-recently-deceased

https://www.sympathymessageideas.com/sympathy-prayers/

https://www.learnreligions.com/dinner-prayers-and-mealtime-blessings-701303

https://connectusfund.org/10-good-opening-prayers-for-funerals

https://elegantmemorials.com/funeral-prayers

Religions

https://www.theregister.co.uk/2006/10/06/the_odd_body_religion/

Saints

https://www.beliefnet.com/faiths/catholic/saints/10-influential-saints-and-their-legends.aspx

https://en.wikipedia.org/wiki/St._Germain_(Theosophy)

Science

Angel particle - https://newatlas.com/angel-particle-own-antiparticle/50579/

Atom - https://en.wikipedia.org/wiki/Atom

https://www.livescience.com/37206-atom-definition.html

Spirit Attachments

https://soulhealer.com/attached-entities-bad-guys-spirit-world/

http://www.entityattachment.com/

Demons

https://en.wikipedia.org/wiki/List_of_demons_in_the_Ars_Goetia

https://en.wikipedia.org/wiki/Classification_of_demons

https://www.mtholyoke.edu/courses/rschwart/hist257/stephwhit/final/hierarchy.html

https://livescifi.tv/2018/07/types-of-demons/

https://kashgar.com.au/blogs/gods-goddesses/a-compendium-of-demons

http://www.supernaturalwiki.com/Demonology

https://greekerthanthegreeks.com/2016/11/good-versus-evil-eternal-conflict.html

https://thisisleviathan.fandom.com/wiki/Seven_Heavenly_Virtues

https://en.wikipedia.org/wiki/Greek_underworld

https://www.beliefnet.com/inspiration/angels/galleries/the-7-archangels-and-their-meanings.aspx

https://en.wikipedia.org/wiki/Voice_of_God

https://www.dummies.com/religion/christianity/catholicism/how-to-pray-the-rosary/

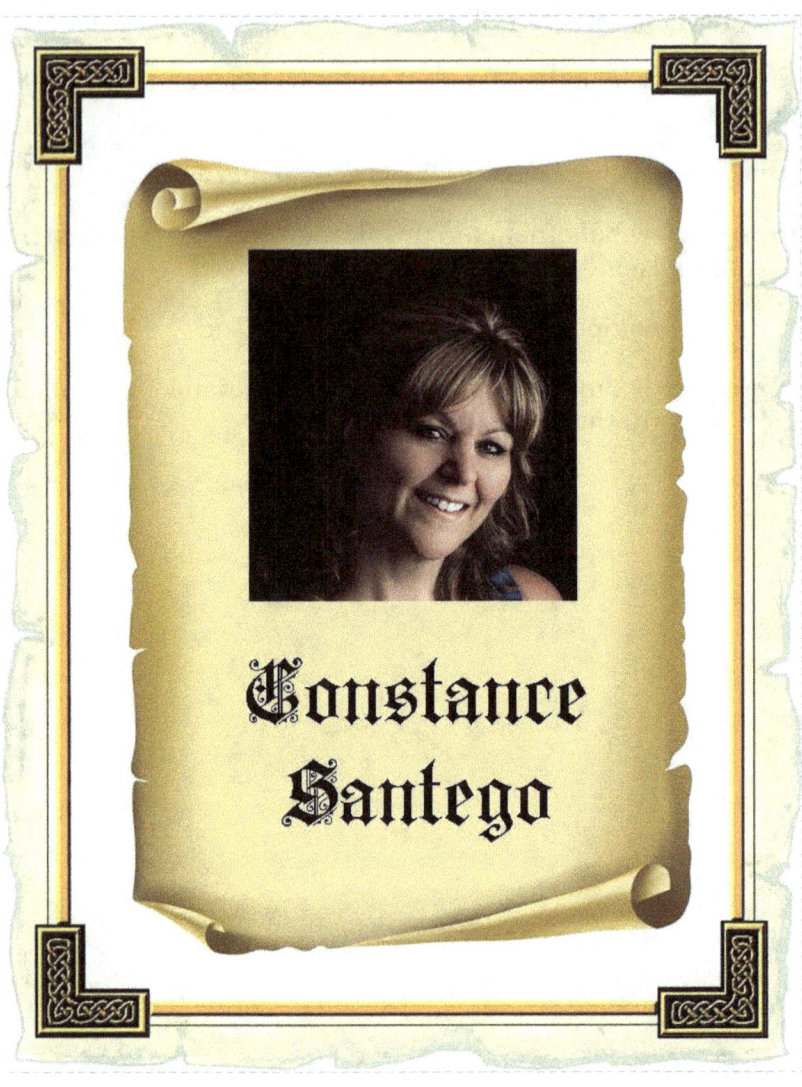

Shift happens...Create magic!
Dream BIGGER!

Constance Santego is a Master Educator and Healer of the Holistic and Spiritual Arts, and Author. She is known for bridging the body, mind, and soul consciousness to transform your dreams into reality.

Constance's background is in business, owning her first company at the age of twenty-seven until her back went out and she had to sell. Learning to heal herself holistically, she gained many, many certificates and diplomas in spirituality and natural healing from amazing schools around the world.

In 1999, she opened a school that became accredited in the holistic arts and ran that until 2012 teaching students from all over the world how to heal themselves and others.

Constance continually strives to advance her knowledge and is currently in the process of attaining her Ph.D. and DOCTORATE in Natural and Integrative Medicine.

The art of healing seems to open a gate to quantum energy, where magic seems to be taking place. But it must be a science since if I can teach others to do what I can do, it can't be imaginary... and if these teachable spiritual gifts are in the Bible, then it has been taught for over two thousand years.

ALSO AVAILABLE

Play the game **Ikona** – Discover Your Virtues and Sins

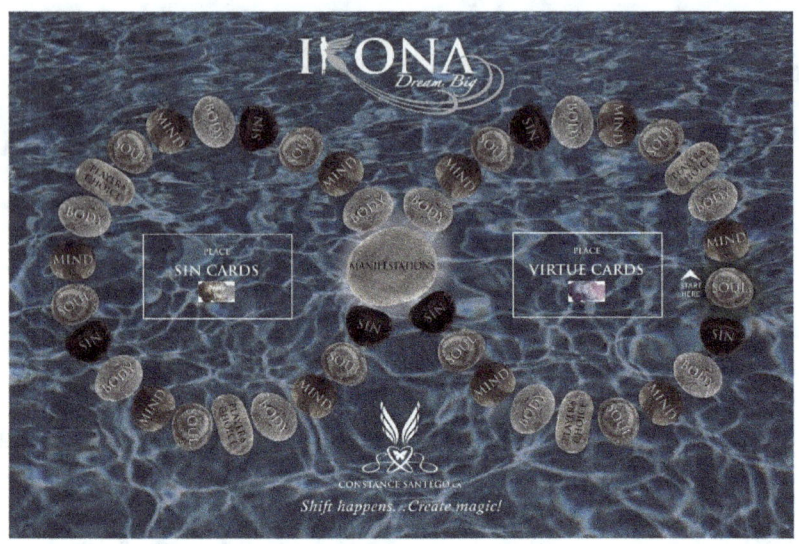

For additional information on

Constance Santego's

wide range of Motivational Products, Coaching Sessions,
Spiritual Retreats,
Live Events and Educational Programs

Go to

www.ConstanceSantego.ca

Follow on Instagram - Constance_Santego &
Facebook - constancesantegoo

Subscribe and receive Free Information and Meditations
on my
YouTube Channel - Constance Santego

www.ingramcontent.com/pod-product-compliance
Lightning Source LLC
Chambersburg PA
CBHW070917080526
44589CB00013B/1337